Behaviour Problems in Developmental Disorders

Behaviour Problems in Developmental Disorders

A *Paediatrician's Guide*

STEWART L. EINFELD

Emeritus Professor, Brain and Mind Centre,
University of Sydney, Australia

MICHAEL McDOWELL

Associate Professor, University of Queensland, Australia

US Consultant

ADRIAN SANDLER

Adjunct Professor, Department of Pediatrics,
University of North Carolina at Chapel Hill, USA

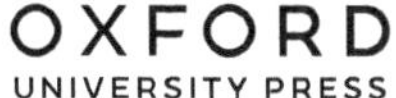

OXFORD
UNIVERSITY PRESS

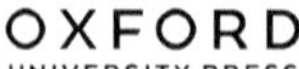

OXFORD
UNIVERSITY PRESS

Great Clarendon Street, Oxford, OX2 6DP,
United Kingdom

Oxford University Press is a department of the University of Oxford.
It furthers the University's objective of excellence in research, scholarship,
and education by publishing worldwide. Oxford is a registered trade mark of
Oxford University Press in the UK and in certain other countries.

Published in the United States of America by Oxford University Press
198 Madison Avenue, New York, NY 10016, United States of America.

British Library Cataloguing in Publication Data

Data available

Library of Congress Control Number: 2025945624

ISBN 978–0–19–289967–5

DOI: 10.1093/med/9780192899675.001.0001

Printed and bound by
CPI Group (UK) Ltd., Croydon, CR0 4YY

The manufacturer's authorised representative in the EU for product safety is
Oxford University Press España S.A. of Parque Empresarial San Fernando de Henares,
Avenida de Castilla, 2 – 28830 Madrid (www.oup.es/en or product.safety@oup.com).
OUP España S.A. also acts as importer into Spain of products made by the manufacturer.

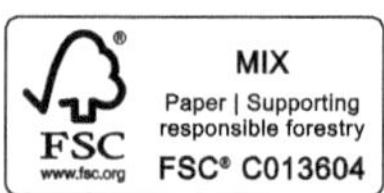

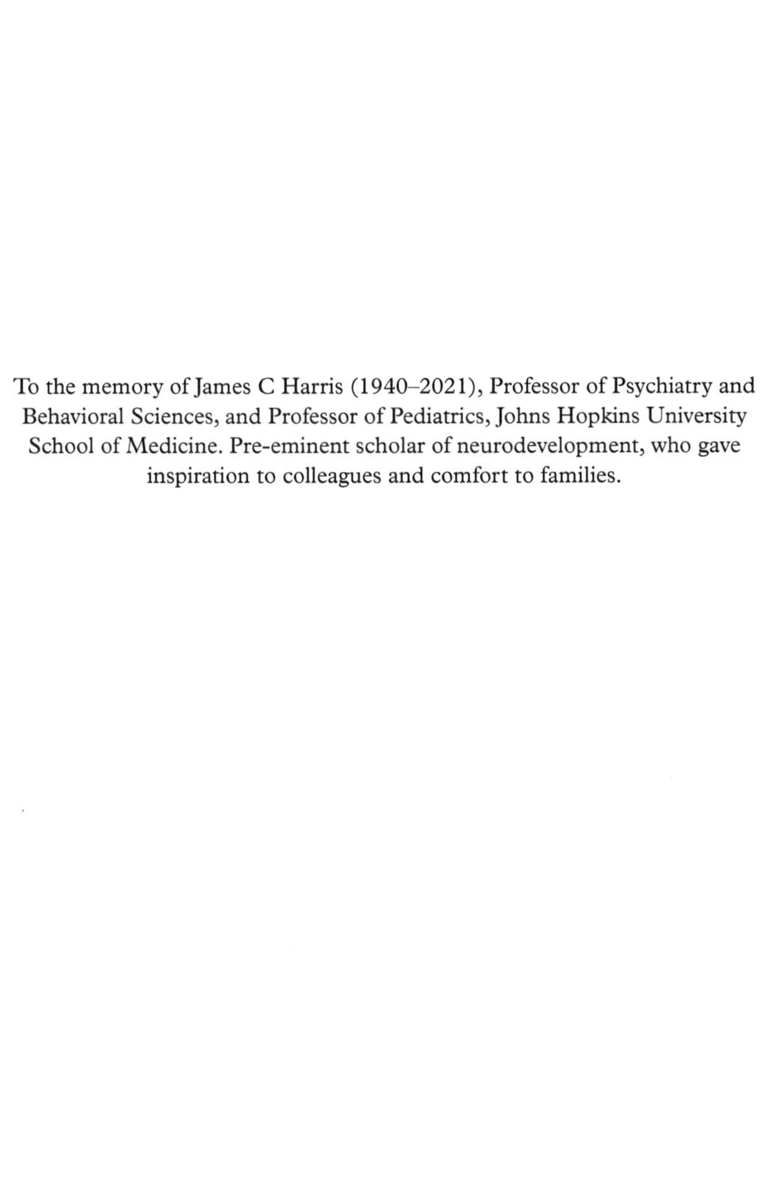

To the memory of James C Harris (1940–2021), Professor of Psychiatry and Behavioral Sciences, and Professor of Pediatrics, Johns Hopkins University School of Medicine. Pre-eminent scholar of neurodevelopment, who gave inspiration to colleagues and comfort to families.

Contents

Acknowledgements

We gratefully acknowledge the contribution of Dr Sylvia Yeung, physician and mother of a boy with severe intellectual disability and autism. Her insights deriving from her lived experience as a parent of a child with disabilities and consumer of specialist paediatric advice has greatly enriched this book.

Declaration of Interest

Professor Einfeld receives royalties from sale of the Developmental Behaviour Checklist, all of which which are donated to child health research.

Foreword

I am a pediatrician with 52 years of experience as a pediatric clinician, educator, researcher, administrator, and editor. As such, I strongly believe that this well-written and referenced book by Stewart Einfeld and Michael McDowell with consultation from Dr. Adrian Sandler should be read by any clinician and perhaps others who care for children. Depending on the country, that might include pediatricians, family medicine physicians, general practitioners, nurse practitioners, physician assistants, and possibly others.

The information provided by a child and adolescent psychiatrist and a developmental pediatrician with input from a consultant behavioural and developmental pediatrician is very important for anyone caring for children. A significant proportion of all children everywhere have developmental and/or behavioural problems. These problems can be the result of birth (difficult deliveries; ingestion of alcohol, drugs, or other toxins by the mother; genetics, etc.); environmental (poor parenting, bullying, exposure to toxins such as lead, etc.), or other problems.

Pediatricians are commonly faced with the task of helping with behaviour problems but are not well prepared from their training for this challenge. This book bridges this gap not only through providing key information but also through providing practical 'how-to' guidance such as conducting family interviews, managing school case conferences, and making reward programmes successful.

No matter their race, creed, gender, or geographic location, all children were created by the same creator and share many gifts and potential or real problems. The work of these experienced authors addresses the many potential and real causes of developmental and behavioural problems of children throughout the world, providing a practical pediatric approach to management.

The authors and consultant are to be lauded for their efforts.

Catherine DeAngelis, MD, MPH
University Distinguished Service Professor,
Professor Emerita, Johns Hopkins Schools of Medicine and Public Health
Editor in Chief Emerita, JAMA

Preface

Why have we written this book?

A large and growing proportion of outpatient (ambulatory, community) general paediatric service workload is now in the clinical area of developmental and behavioural paediatrics. How services are triaged and managed varies by country and system. However the increasing demand for medical services to address child problems of development and behaviour seems to be a universal phenomenon.

The focus of this book is on child behaviour, what children do and say. It is clearly linked to development, mental health, general health, expectations, life circumstances, past experiences, and many other influences. Behaviour may be a problem in its own right (e.g. the child who self-harms or is aggressive to others), or may be the presentation of an underlying problem (bullying at school, abuse, learning difficulties). Often it is both.

As indicated in the book's title, we focus on behaviour problems in children who have developmental disorders, whether suspected, presumed, or diagnosed. It is generally concern about health and development that brings a child into paediatric care. As problems of behaviour are common in this group of children, the focus of paediatric care often extends beyond child health and development to include problematic behaviour.

Training programmes in paediatric medicine emphasize expertise in medical disorders, often at the expense of training in developmental and behavioural paediatric problems. It is not surprising that paediatricians repeatedly rate developmental and behavioural paediatrics as the area of practice for which their training has left them least prepared. As a result, developmental and behavioural clinical problems may not be comfortably managed or even recognized in clinical practice.

This book is written to help paediatricians and other providers of health services to children with disability address this predicament. Despite differences in the nature of paediatric practice across different countries, there is a common challenge when children present with problems of development and behaviour.

Our goal is that the information provided is practical and easily utilized to enhance clinical practice.

About the authors

The book is a collaboration of perspectives, psychiatric and paediatric.

Professor Einfeld is a Child and Adolescent Psychiatrist with a lifelong professional interest in the connections between biology, disability, and behaviour. Over many years, he has provided consultation to paediatricians seeking input on management of children with developmental disabilities and problematic behaviour. This work has given him an understanding of the extra skills and knowledge paediatricians can utilize to aid their patients. Part of this work has been contributing to family support associations for children with various genetic syndromes, including the PraderWilli Syndrome Association of Australia, the Williams Syndrome Association of NSW, and the 22q Foundation of Australia and New Zealand, and others.

Associate Professor McDowell is a Developmental Paediatrician who has worked at an international level to build this area of professional work. He is the founding President of the Australasian Society for Developmental Paediatrics, a body established to support paediatricians in this work. This Society grew rapidly to have more than 900 members across Australia, New Zealand, Singapore, and other South-East Asian countries.

Professor Adrian Sandler is an internationally renowned Developmental-Behavioral Paediatrician and a former President of the Society for Developmental and Behavioral Pediatrics. He has decades of clinical experience as a consultant and he has worked extensively with primary care networks in North Carolina in learning collaboratives to enhance care of children with developmental disabilities. He brings a US perspective to this book.

In our roles as consultants in Child Psychiatry and Developmental Paediatrics, we know that understanding and managing behaviour in this population of children can be complex and challenging. Also, we have come to appreciate the critically important roles of paediatric healthcare providers in meeting this challenge. Our goal in writing this book is to distil key insights, perspectives, and practical approaches from our decades of experience, and share these with readers who are motivated to take better care of their patients.

Who is this book for?

We have written this book for medically trained doctors who assess and manage children in outpatient practice. This practice includes the management of children who have developmental disability and specifically includes management of difficult behaviour in this population of children. This includes, but is not restricted to, the prescription and management of psychotropic medications as part of the strategy for management of problematic behaviour.

In Australia, we follow the English system where paediatrics is a referral speciality. At the same time, there are many primary care generalist doctors (General Practitioners) in Australia whose clinical practice includes a large proportion of child health, including the management of children's behaviour.

The situation differs in the United States where the majority of paediatricians provide primary care services to children. A small number of paediatricians have further specialized (board certified) in Developmental-Behavioral Paediatrics. Most children with disabilities receive primary care from general paediatricians. However, Family Medicine doctors provide approximately 20% of primary care services to children, including many with disability. Nurse Practitioners and Physician Assistants may also provide primary care to children.

Doctors work in a variety of settings and professional structures internationally. They may work as consultants or in primary care. They may be salaried, fee-for-service, or in contracted service. Their work may be geographically bounded or able to take referrals from any location. Regardless of this variation in practice circumstance, we write this book for doctors who provide continuing care for children who have developmental disorders.

Throughout this book we use the term 'paediatrician' as a non-specific term for medical doctors who see children. We understand that in different parts of the world this term conveys different meanings. We are also aware that many doctors who manage children with developmental disorders would not describe themselves as paediatricians. Examples include primary care doctors in Australia, the United Kingdom, and the United States. In the United States this may extend to nurse practitioners and physician assistants who provide ongoing health services to children with disability.

We use the phrase '**developmental paediatrics**' in this book as a non-specific descriptor for this area of work. In different countries this may convey different meanings, particularly regarding clinical problems referenced. In this book we use 'developmental paediatrics' to mean:

- Work undertaken by medically trained doctors.

- Working with children and youth, but not adults.

- Working with clinical problems that impact development, including learning and behaviour. This may range in severity from learning problems in a mainstream classroom through to non-verbal manifestations of intellectual impairment and autism.

- Working from a developmental perspective. This includes management as well as treatment, working across long-term time frames as well as shorter periods of care and working within ecological and biopsychosocial frameworks.

What we have assumed

Clinical practice, knowledge, and skills

When discussing behaviour of children with developmental disorders, we make a number of assumptions regarding the reader's practice, knowledge and skills.

- **Continuing Care of Developmental Disorders**: Following assessment, we assume the reader will take a significant level of responsibility for continuing medical care, including management of associated behavioural problems. For common developmental disorders particularly (e.g. Attention Deficit Hyperactivity Disorder), we assume the reader has the knowledge and skills to undertake medical management (e.g. prescription and management of stimulant medication), guided as appropriate by local practice guidelines.

- **General medicine**: For medical care generally, we assume capacity to assess and manage medical problems, including the medical exploration of possible aetiology (e.g. genetic testing) or confounding issues (e.g. seizures, possible sources of pain, gastrointestinal (GIT) problems) that occur in children who have developmental disorders.

- **Developmental medicine**: For developmental disorders specifically, we assume the reader has the knowledge and training to undertake the assessment necessary to conclude developmental diagnoses, or has the referral resources necessary to address this appropriately for the children they see. This includes local practice guidelines for diagnostic assessment as appropriate. The process may or may not involve referral for specialist and/or other professional input.

Practice circumstances

Practice circumstances vary with regards to how children come to consultation (referral pathways), and the role taken by the paediatrician. This may take place as part of a multidisciplinary team, or as the sole provider.

While recognizing this variation, it is beyond the scope of this book to consider all possible situations. Instead, we will attempt to present information according to guiding principles, relying on clinicians to interpret these in an individualized manner that best fits with their local circumstances.

Age considerations

Young people with developmental disabilities often have behavioural challenges continuing into their twenties that are typical for younger individuals/teenagers. These are included within the age remit of this book.

Scope

As this is intended to be a clinical guidebook, we will not provide comprehensive coverage of child development, mental health, and behaviour. Such information is available through textbooks on the relevant subjects. Suggested textbooks are included where relevant. As a guidebook we take a principles-based approach rather than clinical algorithms. It is up to the clinician to select and apply these as appropriate for individual clinical situations.

We have included clinical cases as example applications of these principles. Three cases thread across all chapters and three additional cases are presented in Chapter 7. All cases represent challenges we see in practice. The names and details do not apply to specific individual cases.

To assist the flow of information, we separate information that may be more detailed and optional in nature from core concepts in the main text. This is differentiated with text boxes as additional reading.

The first two chapters focus on conceptual issues in understanding behaviour in children. Chapter 4 addresses issues of diagnosis and diagnostic formulation at both a conceptual and practical level. Chapters 3 to 6 emphasize practical issues and clinical applications, and Chapter 7 includes several illustrative cases. Throughout the book we have highlighted practice tips and key take-home messages.

Nomenclature

Official taxonomies: Different countries utilize different diagnostic and coding systems, principally the US Diagnostic and Statistical Manual-5 (DSM-5 (1), or the World Health Organization International Classification of Diseases (ICD-11) (2). In the DSM system, making a diagnosis depends on a conjoint assessment of symptoms and functioning, whereas the ICD considers mental disorders separate from attributable impairments (3). Function may be independently characterized, for example, using the International Classification of

Functioning, Disability and Health (ICF) (4). Where diagnostic categorization is utilized in this book we will indicate which system we use to do this.

Developmental Disabilities: According to US Public Law 106-402 developmental disability is defined as a severe, chronic disability in an individual that is attributable to a mental or physical impairment, is manifested before the individual attains age 22, is likely to continue indefinitely, and results in substantial functional limitations in three or more functional areas.

In this book we use the term 'developmental disabilities' to define a set of problems that extend this definition to include a broader range of problems seen in paediatric practice. An example is the child who has Specific Learning Disability who has functional problem on one area only. Specific syndromes and disorders are discussed in Chapter 6 along with their functional and behavioural consequences and associations. We also clarify the term 'developmental syndromes' in Chapter 6. The range of severity is considered in Chapter 1 and functional domains in Chapter 2. Some mental health disorders may not be considered as developmental disabilities, however we have included these also in Chapter 6 as they often co-occur with developmental disabilities and impact on child behaviour.

Language of behaviour: In Chapter 1 we discuss properties of behaviour that make it a problem for the child. In referencing this set of behaviours we use a variety of terms. These terms include: mental health problems, psychopathology, problem behaviours, difficult behaviour, challenging behaviours, behaviours of concern, and others. We use these terms interchangeably as descriptors. We do not use these terms to imply different theories of causation. Included in this set are emotional problems whose behavioural expression may be internalizing or avoidant because we do not wish to overlook the child who is suffering without causing disruption to others.

Non-judgemental intent: Terminology in the clinical area of child development and behaviour is not straightforward. A fundamental principle with the terminology used in this book is that terms used do not imply value judgement. We hold firm to the view that all children are of equal value, regardless of their developmental capacity or behaviour.

Description of children with diagnosed disorders: Beyond categorization systems, there is variation regarding how diagnostic language is used in clinical communications. For criteria-based diagnoses, when we use diagnostic language in this book (e.g. 'the child has …'), we recognize this is a shorthand convenience in place of the more accurate, but linguistically cumbersome 'the child has been assessed as meeting diagnostic criteria for …'.

Disabled child or child with a disability: We refer to the child who has, for example, a diagnosed Autism Spectrum Disorder rather than the Autistic child. We consider this to be respectful to the child and consistent with medical thinking (e.g. the child who has Systemic Lupus Erythematosus). We recognize that some but not all adolescents and adults may prefer to be identified with their diagnosis by being called an 'autistic person' or a 'deaf person'.

Typically developing children: Various terms are in use to describe children without disability. These include: typically developing, regular, average, neurotypical, normally developing. In this book we have chosen to use the term 'typically developing'.

Families: We acknowledge that families are constituted of a broad range of different people, and in multiple possible arrangements. While the term 'parents' generally refers to mothers and fathers, we extend this to include adults performing the carer parenting role. It may mean a male and female adult, or persons of any combination of genders. It may also mean grandparents, other relatives, legal guardians, or caregivers in the parenting role.

Gender language: Rather than the potentially cumbersome 'he/she' and 'his/her' we have chosen to use gender neutral pronouns such as 'they' and 'their'.

References

(1) American Psychiatric Association. Diagnostic and statistical manual of mental disorders: DSM-5. 5th edition. Arlington, VA: American Psychiatric Association; 2013. 947 p.

(2) International Classification of Diseases (ICD) [Internet]. [cited 16 May 2022]. Available from: https://www.who.int/standards/classifications/classification-of-diseases. Published in 2022.

(3) Üstün B, Kennedy C. What is 'functional impairment'? Disentangling disability from clinical significance. World Psychiatry. 2009 Jun;8(2):82–5.

(4) International Classification of Functioning, Disability and Health (ICF) [Internet]. [cited 23 Oct 2023]. Available from: https://www.who.int/standards/classifications/international-classification-of-functioning-disability-and-health. Published in 2001.

Abbreviations

The following abbreviations are used. In cases where additional abbreviations are used, they will be written out in full along with the abbreviation at the first instance.

ABA	Applied Behaviour Analysis
A-B-C	Antecedents-Behaviour-Consequences
ABC	Aberrant Behaviour Checklist
ADHD	Attention Deficit Hyperactivity Disorder
AFO	Ankle Foot Orthosis
ARFID	Avoidant/Restrictive Food Intake Disorder
ASD	Autism Spectrum Disorder
ASEBA	Achenbach System of Empirical Behaviour Measurement
BMI	Body Mass Index
CBCL	Child Behaviour Checklist
CBIT	Comprehensive Behavioural Intervention for Tics
CBT	Cognitive Behaviour Therapy
CD	Conduct Disorder
CP	Cerebral Palsy
CPK	creatine phosphokinase
CTOPP	Comprehensive Test of Phonological Processing
DBC	Developmental Behaviour Checklist
DCD	Developmental Coordination Disorder
DC-LD	Diagnostic Criteria-Learning Disorders
DMDD	Disruptive Mood Dysregulation Disorder
DM-ID	Diagnostic Manual—Intellectual Disability
DRA	Differential Reinforcement of Alternative Behaviours
DRO	Differential Reinforcement of Other Behaviours
DSM-5	Diagnostic and Statistical Manual, 5th Edition
DSM-ID-2	Diagnostic Manual—Intellectual Disability, 2nd Edition
EEG	Electroencephalogram
ESDM	Early Start Denver Model

FASD	Fetal Alcohol Spectrum Disorder
FAST	Functional Assessment Screening Tool
FTC	Functional Communication Training
GAD	Generalized Anxiety Disorder
GIT	gastrointestinal
GMFCS	Gross Motor Function Classification System
GOF	Goodness of Fit
HRT	Habit Reversal Therapy
ICD-11	International Classification of Diseases, 11th Edition
ICF	International Classification of Functioning, Disability and Health
ID	Intellectual Disability
IDEA	Individuals with Disabilities Education Act (United States)
LHRH	Luteinizing-hormone releasing hormone
NICE	National Institute for Health and Care Excellence
OCD	Obsessive-Compulsive Disorder
ODD	Oppositional Defiant Disorder
OT	Occupational Therapy
PBS	Positive Behaviour Support
prn	pro re nata
PTSD	Post-traumatic Stress Disorder
PWS	Prader-Willi Syndrome
RAD	Reactive Attachment Disorder
RRBs	Restrictive and Repetitive Behaviours
SCARED	Screen for Childhood Anxiety and Related Disorders
SDQ	Strengths and Difficulties Questionnaire
SIB	Self-Injurious Behaviours
SLD	Specific Learning Disorder
SNRI	Serotonin-Norepinephrine Reuptake Inhibitor
SS	Scaled Score
SSBP	Society for the Study of Behavioural Phenotypes
SSRI	Selective Serotonin Reuptake Inhibitor
UPD	uniparental disomy
VCSF	Velocardiofacial syndrome
WISC-V	Wechsler Intelligence Scale for Children, 5th Edition

1

A paediatric perspective

Managing behaviour problems is deeply rewarding. Like a complex surgical procedure, it takes time.

In our roles as consultants in Child Psychiatry and Developmental Paediatrics, we know that understanding and managing behaviour for children with developmental disorders can be complex and challenging. Paediatricians understand a child's developmental capabilities and perspectives and are skilled in explanation and advocacy. They are attuned to the ethical complexities of caring for children, especially children with disabilities. The paediatric perspective appreciates and works within context such as family, friends, and school. These skills and perspectives are particularly important when children are not able to speak for themselves.

Developmental disability and child behaviour

Problems of development and behaviour are common in paediatric medical practice. They have been shown to comprise more than 50% of both new and review consultations in Australia (1). The range of developmental disorders is wide. At one end are problems experienced by children able to attend mainstream classes, participating in regular curriculum. Such high-prevalence problems affect self-control (e.g. Attention Deficit Hyperactivity Disorder), learning and communication (e.g. Specific Learning Disorders, Language Disorders), social function (e.g. mild Autism Spectrum Disorders (ASDs)), emotional well-being (e.g. Anxiety Disorders), and motor control (e.g. Developmental Coordination Disorder).

At the other end of this range are problems that necessitate individualized care and educational supports. How such supports are provided may vary, from classroom inclusion models through to more restrictive special educational environments. This level of individualized adaptation is often necessary for children with moderate to severe Intellectual Disability (ID), Cerebral Palsy, and ASDs.

All across this range, the likelihood of associated behavioural problems is higher than typically developing children (2), comprising a significant proportion of clinical practice (3). Supports required at school may be determined as much by the associated behaviours as by the individual child's learning needs (4).

Understanding a child's functioning, disability, and health are of central importance in understanding and managing their behaviour. There are several ways of doing this. The International Classification of Functioning, Disability and Health (ICF) (5). The ICF is closely tied to the International Classification of Diseases (ICD-11), the current global standard for classification of diseases. The ICF recognizes the important effects of environmental barriers and facilitators and associated health factors in understanding an individual's functional capacities, activities, and participation in daily life.

The approach of this book is similar to the ICD/ICF model but focuses specifically on behaviour problems, rather than the broader ICF focus on function, activities, and participation. We use a formulation structure as the basis both for understanding the causes of behaviour and for planning management. As with ICF, this integrates health, disability, and relevant environmental factors.

Each child is only able to manage behaviour according to their developmental capacities, determined in large part by brain function. These directly influence a child's comprehension, communication, social understanding, and self-control. Behaviour is further influenced by each child's physiology (e.g. sleep, fatigue, pain), temperament, mood state, and mental health, all within the historical context of the child's life experience. Beyond developmental capacities, behaviour is influenced by the child's world, their safety, and the degree to which expectations are adapted and appropriate for that child. These considerations comprise the bio-psycho-social model used in this book to understand the multiple contributions to child behaviour. Behaviour could be considered a 'final common pathway' for all these influencing factors.

This book focuses on the needs of the paediatrician providing clinical care. Although of great importance, this book does not address public health and general advocacy aspects of developmental disabilities and accompanying behaviour problems. This includes access to services and preventive strategies such as reducing community exposure to lead poisoning, foetal alcohol, and trauma from wars.

Ethical issues

Care of children with disability, particularly management of problem behaviour, is an area where clinical practice and guidance are built on a foundation of ethical principles. Paediatricians working in this area necessarily do so within ethical frameworks that apply to all children (such as the UN Convention on the Rights of the Child (6)), specific to children with disability (such as the Global Report on Children with Developmental Disabilities (7)), and those written for paediatricians (e.g. (8)). In some countries and states there are statutory requirements related to ethical care of children with developmental disabilities.

Models of disability

A fundamental ethical consideration is how disability is understood. The 'Social Model' of disability is a framework that is often discussed in contrast to the 'Medical Model'. Both models contribute in a beneficial way to understanding and helping children, yet this dichotomy may fracture services and collaboration between professionals (9).

The Social Model has grown in response to what is perceived as individual devaluation and dehumanization associated with deficit-based thinking and practice that is sometimes ascribed to the Medical Model. In a deficit paradigm, sometimes referred to currently as 'ableism', individuals are considered to have problems that need to be fixed, implying that they are of lower value or worth because of their developmental problems.

The approach of this book is that children have full value, worth, and humanity as they are. All children are defined by their humanity, actions, interests, abilities, and passions—not by their disability.

The struggle for children with disabilities arises in two ways. First, the world may not be adapted for their needs. Where possible, care begins with addressing this adaptation. Second, brain dysfunction can directly cause impairment which has direct consequences for quality of life, participation, and capacity to learn/develop. In childhood particularly, however, impairments are not fixed. Neuroplasticity enables the benefits of interventions to be amplified over time. The earlier the intervention, the longer the child is able to benefit.

How should we think of interventions to manage behaviour and build capacity while respecting differences?

1. **Child-centric, child-affirming**: Ensure every decision is justifiable towards making life better for the child. At every stage the child's interests, capacities, wishes, and perspectives are heard and incorporated as appropriate.

2. **Affirmation and respect**: Choose language that respects the whole child, minimizing communication that may be understood as defining and judging children by their impairments and diagnoses.

3. **Adaptation and support**: Begin intervention with goodness-of-fit adaptations. These aim to change the expectations and support within a child's world so that they align with the child's capacities. The goal is that the child lives and grows in an adapted world, able to meet demands and expectations, maximizing their capacity to function independently.

4. **Intervention and skill-building**: All children receive interventions to enhance their development and learning. For children with disabilities, rather than communicating these interventions as remediating deficits, they need to be individualized capacity building steps towards a more functional, enjoyable, and successful future—fundamentally no different from any other child.

5. **Freedom of choice**: The decision to intervene with a behaviour problem is a decision of the parents and, to the extent possible, the child. It is not fundamentally a decision of the paediatrician. There are explicit circumstances, however, where the paediatrician is obliged to intervene. These include situations where abuse may be occurring or there is a serious safety risk for the child, for example serious intent to self-harm. In both cases, the intervention process is managed by local regulations.

In this book specific ethical matters are addressed in the chapters where they are most relevant:

◆ Later in this chapter the properties of behaviour that make intervention appropriate are discussed. Regarding behaviour more generally, the goal across this book is to understand what the child is communicating and intervene where necessary in a way that optimizes quality of life, participation, and development as well as reducing harm and distress for the child.

◆ Chapters 3 (Assessment), 4 (Diagnosis and Diagnostic Formulation), and 5 (Management) consider the balance of acceptance and intervention. These chapters are written from a bio-psycho-social perspective, with the child's and family's voices and well-being at the centre. Chapter 5 also touches on the tensions that may arise when the principle of beneficence (doing what is considered beneficial for the patient) is not necessarily aligned with the principle of autonomy (respecting the patient's choice). Such tensions may be eased through shared decision-making.

◆ Chapter 5 (Management) addresses the specific questions of restrictive practices. With regards to behaviour these include physical as well as medical (pharmacological) restraint.

> ## Practice tip: Think globally, practice locally
>
> Paediatricians working with children who have disability should be familiar with relevant general ethical guidelines. It is necessary, however, to know of and work within local regulations that govern ethical care of children with disabilities.

The medical perspective

In this book we approach child behaviour from a standard medical perspective. In general medicine, medical thinking works through a sequence beginning with history (symptoms) → physical examination (signs) → differential diagnosis → investigations → diagnosis → treatment → treatment-related outcomes. These skills are grounded in knowledge of normal function (e.g. anatomy, physiology), problematic function (e.g. pathology), and discrete clinical conditions (clinical presentation, aetiology, natural history, and prognosis).

This process is recursive. The skilled clinician uses intervention expectations to monitor progress. If outcomes are not as expected, hypotheses can be revised regarding causal processes and what needs to be do3ne.

What we have observed in clinical practice is that many of these steps are sometimes bypassed when doctors evaluate and manage problematic child behaviour. A common 'short circuit' pathway may begin with the behaviour, move to diagnosis (e.g. ADHD), and then to diagnosis-determined treatment (e.g. choice of medication). Limited training in child behaviour makes it difficult to work systematically through the full set of clinical steps.

All steps of standard medical thinking are appropriate for behaviour problems. We will take as an example a child presenting with abdominal pain. In Table 1.1, we compare the knowledge and clinical skills for managing abdominal pain with those for behaviour problems. The final column indicates where in this book the issues are addressed.

Table 1.1 Abdominal pain compared with a behaviour problem in a child with a developmental disorder. The following table is intended to show that behaviour problems can be approached using the same model as in internal medicine, with which paediatricians are familiar.

	Abdominal Pain	Behaviour Problem	Chapter
Possible mechanisms	Injury, obstruction, inflammation, infection, metabolic abnormality, malignancy	Child: developmental, self-control, mood instability. Environment: abuse, trauma, unachievable expectations	Chapter 2
Assessment	Assess the child: History Examination Investigations guided by differential diagnosis	Describe the behaviour, Assess the child, the family, and the child's environment for causal factors	Chapter 3
Putting information together	Make a diagnosis	Understand how multiple contributing factors fit together (formulation)	Chapter 4
		Understand contribution of particular disorders and syndromes	Chapter 6
Management	Medical and non-medical treatments and supports	Behaviour management; therapy with the child; changes to the environment; medication; review/strategy revision	Chapter 5

The time challenge

Assessing and managing behaviour takes time. While some situations may be straightforward, many are complex. More time is needed to understand and manage behaviour than a routine consultation for asthma or eczema. Consulting circumstances vary. Available supporting resources from other professions also vary. Different systems may limit numbers of services able to be provided for each child or require discharge at particular ages. Clinicians adapt as fits their situation, for example:

- Collecting information prior to the first visit (e.g. questionnaires, assessments, review by allied health professionals)

- Organizing longer consultation times for complex cases

- Utilizing efficient methods of documentation

- Arranging sets of sequential visits

- Referring out components of necessary assessment and/or management within a multidisciplinary group

It is in the doctor's (and the child's) interest to find a way of allocating time and activities that enables good clinical practice. This increases the probability of 'getting it right' from the outset, setting up a formulation and management approach that enables revision of hypothesis and strategy if initial approaches are not successful. Spending the necessary time from the outset builds trust, involving families and other providers in the formulation and management plan. Without this, doctors risk finding themselves in a repetitive cycle of prescription and referral.

In summary, substantial time and work is usually necessary to manage difficult behaviour successfully. In this book we offer concepts and principles. We trust individual doctors to find ways to apply these principles in the individual circumstances of their practice.

> ## Practice tip: Time is necessary for success
>
> Assessing and managing behaviour problems requires more time than is needed for general physical health problems. A rushed approach to behaviour problems is less likely to lead to effective management.

Child behaviour

Behaviour as clinical information

As clinical information, behaviour has properties both in common with, as well as extending beyond traditional medical symptoms and signs. The following are some examples of these properties:

- **Behaviour is observable:** It is what might be observed and heard in the office or in a video clip.

- **A sequence over time:** It is a sequence of action that changes over time. It may be considered to have time boundaries, with a beginning, middle, and end.

- **State dependent**: The clinical assessment of a child varies if they are febrile, breathless, or fatigued. Similarly, child behaviour depends on the child's state, for example tired, angry, feeling anxious or threatened.

- **Environment and context dependent**: A lump or a rash are generally consistent across environments. By contrast, behaviour may vary depending on the environment the child is in. Such contextual variation provides information regarding the extent to which behaviour is biologically driven, or what situational triggers influence the behaviour.

- **Interpreted within developmental, social, and cultural expectations**: Just as child growth parameters are interpreted by child age and gender, a developmental and cultural context of normal behaviour is necessary to interpret behaviours. An example is avoiding eye contact, which may be appropriate for the child's culture.

- **Capacity for intention**: Children do not choose to have fever, rash, cough, or short stature. By contrast, hypotheses of intention may be part of the description of behaviour.

Describing behaviour

In medical practice, clinical phenomena (pain, lump, rash) are defined in a standardized way. In a similar manner, the description of behaviour can be standardized. The more accurate the characterization of behaviour, the more successful clinical intervention is likely to be.

Practice tip: Primary vs secondary (interpreted) data

It is important to separate the description of the behaviour from interpretations of the behaviour. The behaviour is literally what would be seen and heard in a video. Any description of the behaviour introduces potential biases of the reporter or observer.

1. The clinician should consider possible biases in reporting and observing behaviour, including their own possible biases.

2. Presumptions of *why* the child may have acted as they did should be clearly separated.

Since behaviour occurs as an interaction between the child and their immediate world, a full definition of behaviour includes context, including location, time, people present, etc. From the context information there are three useful observations relevant to understanding behaviour (discussed in greater detail in Chapter 3):

- **Precipitating**: What sets the behaviour in motion, for example the child not getting what they want, non-preferred activities/demands, or something unexpected

- **Perpetuating**: Once the behaviour has started, what serves to keep it going, for example a response that is loud and angry, or experienced by the child as accusatory.

- **Palliating**: Once the behaviour has started, what serves to settle it down, for example a gentle, trusted person providing diversion, or strategies to soothe the child.

We note two common obstacles to gaining accurate characterization of behaviour.

1. **Interpretation.** We would not generally rely on history that a blood pressure was high or blood sugar low, instead making that determination for ourselves, or using sources of known reliability such as lab reports. When communicating behaviour, however, history from observers often comes pre-packaged as interpretation. An example is the report that a child has been defiant or angry. This is not the same as what the child says and does. It overlooks the environmental factors that trigger and perpetuate that behaviour. It attributes intention to the behaviour.

2. **Perspectives.** How behaviour is observed, remembered, and interpreted is individual. Different observers may have different recollections, as well as interpretations, of the behaviour. This can make it difficult for the paediatrician to determine which behaviours are actually occurring.

Assessment strategies we have found useful to describe behaviour, and manage these potential hurdles, are discussed further in Chapter 4.

Is the behaviour a problem appropriate for medical care?

Having sufficient objective information about the child's behaviour, the next recommended step is to be clear as to why this problem is appropriate for medical care.

In the context of this disorder, normal behavioural variation may be appropriately managed by parents and school. Behaviour outside this normal range that is associated with family and child psychological struggles may be considered the domain of psychological/behavioural health services. Behaviour that breaks the law is the domain of the criminal justice system. In what circumstances is it appropriate for the paediatrician to become involved?

Families have a relationship with the paediatrician and are likely to seek help from their doctor for their child's behaviour. The understanding and management of child behaviour may require knowledge and understanding of the child's underlying developmental disorder. Also, medical treatment such as psychotropic medication may be required for managing the condition.

Behaviour as a problem for the child

In addition to these practical reasons, assessment and management by the paediatrician can be appropriate clinically when the behaviour is a **problem for the child**. Understanding why it is a problem for the child also guides management.

Voice: The behaviour may be the child's 'voice'. A child's behaviour may be the expression of an underlying problem that needs to be understood and addressed. This is particularly important for children who are less able to communicate and advocate for themselves:

- The behaviour indicates that the child is suffering, for example very anxious, unwell, or in pain

- The behaviour may arise because the child is not able to understand, or to do what is expected of them

- The behaviour is an adaptation to problematic circumstances, such as domestic violence or bullying

Direct harm: The behaviour may be directly harmful to the child, for example, when:

- The child hurts themselves

- The behaviour results in psychological harm to the child (e.g. they are blamed for behaviour they cannot help)

- The behaviour interferes with or limits the child's learning and development

- The behaviour interferes with or limits the child's capacity for participation in, and enjoyment of day-to-day life activities

Internalized harm: Behaviour may indicate the child is suffering, even though the behaviour itself is not overtly problematic, for example when:

- The child withdraws from social opportunity

- The child 'disconnects' with reduced participation

- The child's desire and associated effort in developmental activities (e.g. learning, sports) diminishes

Harm to others: The behaviour may be harmful to other people, animals, or objects, for example, when:

- The child hurts others

- In response to the child's behaviour, others feel very upset or threatened

- The behaviour limits learning and development of others (e.g. disruptive behaviour in the classroom)

- The behaviour limits participation by others (e.g. the family cannot go out into the community as they may wish)

- The behaviour harms animals

- The behaviour damages property

Harm in interpretation: Finally, reported behaviour may not be problematic in itself, but problems arise because of how others interpret and respond. If observer expectations are not appropriate for a child's capacity, it is the job of the doctor to conduct an assessment and draw their own conclusions. For example:

- Oppositional/defiant behaviour may be normal for the child's developmental level

- Inattentive/impulsive behaviour may be appropriate for context, developmental level, or cause no harm to the child

- Lack of participation or socially withdrawn behaviour may have many causes

- Aggressive, fight/flight behaviour may be appropriately self-defensive

We note that multiple observers often have different interpretations and beliefs regarding a child's behaviour. In order to understand fully what is causing the behaviour, it is usually necessary to understand what all the key stakeholders observe and believe regarding a child's behaviour.

How this book is structured

The next chapter discusses foundation knowledge and key concepts regarding behaviour in children who have developmental problems.

- **Chapter 2—Causes of Behaviour Problems.** This chapter provides a summary overview of child and environmental factors that contribute to child behaviour problems.

- **Chapter 3—Assessment.** This includes assessment of the child, the family, and gathering information more widely (e.g. from schools).

- **Chapter 4—Diagnosis and Formulation.** This chapter discusses the theory of diagnosis and formulation. Diagnosis alone is often insufficient with regards to informing both the cause and management strategy for child behaviour. We propose a formulation model of organizing diagnostic information for behaviour that combines relevant bio-psycho-social information with the time structure of behavioural episodes (before, during, after). We offer an adapted 5-P model as an efficient structure to achieve this (10).

- **Chapter 5—Management.** In addition to medical treatments (particularly psychotropic medication), this chapter addresses non-pharmacological interventions the doctor may initiate, and a basic understanding of interventions undertaken by other professions (sufficient for the doctor to understand and work alongside these).

- **Chapter 6—Syndromes.** This chapter discusses the application of previous chapters to specific clinical syndromes. These are grouped as Genetic, Epileptic, Developmental, Teratogenic, and Mental Health.

- **Chapter 7—Clinical Case Examples.** In each of the Chapters 1 to 6 we present brief case vignettes with associated discussion points to illustrate key issues from each chapter. In Chapter 7 we provide additional cases for readers to review. These diverse cases reinforce the concepts of the book and may be additional helpful in teaching these concepts to others.

Chapter summary

This chapter considers the important role paediatricians take in the management of behaviour problems with children with disability.

- There is a high incidence of behaviour problems among children with developmental disorders.

- Behaviour is a problem when it causes hurt and/or distress to the child or others, and when it impairs the child's function and development.

- When caring for children with disability, the paediatrician has an important role in understanding and managing associated behaviour problems as well as functional impairments.

- Paediatric intervention is built on an ethical framework.

- Objective data is much better than information already interpreted by others.

- Using objective information, behaviour problems can be understood and managed with the structures, methodology, and tools of standard medical practice.

- This work generally takes more time than outpatient medical care.

Appendix 1.1—Case examples

After each chapter we will present three cases and discussion prompts. The discussion prompts reflect issues raised in the chapter. The cases will continue through the book. In Chapter 7 three further cases are presented, each raising different issues regarding the assessment and management of challenging behaviour in children who have developmental disorders.

Case 1. Jack

Jack provides an example of behaviour in the context of multiple simultaneous contributing risk factors, each of similar impact. These include his developmental impairments, family, and school factors.

Jack is a 9-year-old boy seen because of aggressive and defiant behaviour, worsening over time. He is brought to see you by his foster mother. Jack has been in and out of foster home care since the age of 18 months. His current placement is stable. His foster parents intend to care for him long term.

Jack presents as socially engaged and personable. A recent multidisciplinary assessment found Jack met criteria for Foetal Alcohol Spectrum Disorder (FASD). In the same assessment a diagnosis of ADHD was made. He did not meet criteria for Autistic Spectrum Disorder. From this assessment it is known he has problems with:

- **Learning:** His measured IQ is 74. His reading is three years behind grade expectation, maths one to two years behind.

- **Language:** Jack's expressive skills are impaired (Scaled Score (SS) on standardized language assessment 66), and receptive skills borderline (SS 72).

- **Executive control:** He has been diagnosed with ADHD and is treated with long-acting methylphenidate.

- **Emotional control:** Jack has disproportionate responses to perceived threat.

- **Motor coordination:** Jack meets criteria for Developmental Coordination Disorder.

Discussion

What do you need to know about Jack's behaviour in order to understand it?

The current description of Jack's behaviour (aggressive, defiant, and worsening over time) is interpreted through the perspective of his foster mother. In clinical practice we seek to form independent opinion regarding presenting symptoms and signs, to understand the behaviour objectively rather than relying on the interpretation of others.

We need to become aware of the problem behaviours as if viewed on CCTV. What specific behaviours would be observed? What would be heard? Does he hit foster parents, students, or teachers? Does he disrupt the class? How did these behaviours begin, persist, and resolve? Assessment aims to understand behaviour at this level of specificity. Building on this understanding, we can then explore the frequency, contextual variation, and history of the behaviour.

In what possible ways is Jack's behaviour harmful to himself, and harmful to others?

This question concerns the reasons we should be involved in Jack's care. It is our goal to prevent or minimize harm. There are several potential harms for Jack. His behaviour may interfere with his learning, development, and social relationships. His behaviour may impact the way others understand him and are willing to help him. His behaviour leads to feedback that Jack assimilates over time, solidifying negative beliefs about himself that may influence future choices.

There are several potential harms for others. Jack's behaviour may include hitting and threatening. There is possible harm to his parents, their confidence, and their optimism. There may be harm in the classroom to other children from his disruptive behaviour.

What do you see as your role within the network of people involved in Jack's care?

As a paediatrician, you should consider Jack's general health and lifestyle. He may need help, for example, with sleep. In addition to the medical management of ADHD, there may be a case for using medication to help Jack's emotional control.

Beyond medication, there is a potential role for the paediatrician in helping others understand what is going on, advocating for necessary support, guiding them about successful strategies, working together to evaluate outcomes, and changing strategies as needed. Finally, you may have an important role talking with Jack himself, helping him understand, accept, and help himself.

Case 2. Jade

Jade is a 14-year-old girl in her second year of high school. When youth present as closed, disrespectful, and intentional, it is tempting to collude with others around a subtle 'blame the child' orientation. Jade's behaviour, however, is her way of communicating that she cannot manage life as she currently experiences it.

You first saw Jade three years ago because of emotional outbursts, at which time you made a diagnosis of mild ASD and noted her strong intelligence and language capacity. You have not seen her since then.

Jade presents again because of problem behaviour. Her family reports Jade's behaviour initially settled down, however it has worsened since early high school. She is described as more angry and non-compliant at home, with increasing school avoidance, currently attending school only half the time.

Jade's parents clearly love her and are committed to helping her. They are worried about the impact of her behaviour on their younger son who is described as 'sensitive'.

Discussion

Before proceeding with consideration of possible causes and management strategy, what do you need to know about Jade's behaviour itself?

School avoidance: You need accurate information regarding attendance that includes days, and times within the day. What does she do when she is home? What are her sleep habits? What is known about her use of electronic media?

Behaviour at home: You need descriptions not only of what Jade does (e.g. shouting, obscene language, locking herself in her room) but also the circumstances (what started this), how it is managed (who said what, what did Jade do in response), contextual variation (what Mum does, what dad does, how the brother responds), and how it resolves.

How might the behaviour cause harm to Jade herself?
How might it cause harm to others?

School avoidance at this stage of her educational journey is clearly harmful to academic achievement. The achievement gap may widen over time.

Jade's adaptive behaviour at home is creating a growing problem for her generally. As her sleep cycle becomes more 'out of sync' with school days, as her screen-based escape behaviours increase, the challenge of rehabilitation becomes correspondingly harder.

Psychologically, Jade is not learning how to cope with stress. She is reinforcing an avoidance strategy that may become habitual and fixed. Beneath this behaviour her self-concept and mental health are likely to be worsening, leading to greater apprehension and resistance to effective strategies.

Her family is suffering in many ways. This includes the marriage, family finances (her mother cannot work full time), the confidence and optimism of both her parents, and the well-being of her younger brother.

Do you consider management of Jade's behaviour to be a valid role for the paediatrician? If so, how does your contribution fit within the network of care?

Diagnosis and medication are unlikely to alter this pattern of maladaptive behaviour substantially, but these problems are likely to be too challenging for either the family or school to manage unassisted. The paediatrician has an important role that includes communication with all key players, a shared way of understanding the problem (based on Diagnostic Formulation), a management plan with step-by-step goals, and the coordination of strategies to achieve those goals.

Are there any ethical issues?

At 14 years of age, Jade is no longer a child, but she is not yet an autonomous adult able to run her own life. It is important for the paediatrician to hear her point of view and manage privacy of information through individualized discussion and explicit contracting. Her growing autonomy needs to be respected; her perspectives on her diagnosis and treatment are important and predictive regarding outcomes. At the same time, it is necessary to balance care of Jade with the needs of her parents and siblings.

Case 3. Alfred

Alfred is a 5-year-old boy with Down syndrome and moderate ID. We included him for several reasons:

1. The cause of his behaviour is uncertain. There are unresolved questions such as parents with different perspectives and concerns about possible abuse.

2. In addition to different perspectives, both parents do not understand Alfred's developmental disability and each has unrealistic expectations.

3. The case illustrates the importance of follow-up and continuity—how family and environmental circumstances may change over time, and how emerging understanding as well as maturity may lead to improvement in this child's behaviour.

His GP refers Alfred to you because of increasing behaviour problems. He has a long history of hyperactive and disruptive behaviour that is a challenge both in preschool and at home. He refuses to participate in tasks and activities in his self-contained class, quickly escalating to throwing things, screaming, and hitting teachers and peers. The school wants him medicated. His GP has tried unsuccessfully to assist Alfred's parents in accessing behaviour therapy. Alfred's father may have unrealistic expectations of Alfred. There is a background of marital conflict. Also, a positive family history of ADHD and substance abuse is noted in his older brother and father.

Alfred is seen in the clinic with his mother and father. He is active and impulsive in the playroom, but refuses the check-in vital signs, falling to the floor, yelling, and trying to hit the nurse. He screams 'No!' and communicates in one- and two-word phrases ('Mummy go'). His mother looks helpless and depressed. His father grabs Alfred firmly by the arms and shouts 'Stop, Alfred! Listen to the nurse!' but the outburst continues. His mother apologizes for his behaviour, and his father quickly says to her, 'You need to be more strict with him.'

Discussion

What challenges do you see in your role as paediatrician in this consultation?

You are faced with several clinical challenges, including:

1. building a therapeutic alliance

2. understanding the causes of Alfred's behaviour

3. managing Alfred's escalation to 'fight and flight' aggression when demands are made

4. reconciling the different perspectives of Alfred's mother and father

5. providing guidance regarding their responses to his behaviour

6. sensitively beginning to probe the marital conflict.

What ethical issues are raised in this consultation?

Alfred's case raises several ethical questions. Does his father's behaviour cross that threshold of suspected abuse, and how should we most helpfully manage this in the clinic? Although clearly a challenge to his caregivers and teachers, how is Alfred's behaviour a problem for him? Would prescribing medication in an effort to make him more compliant necessarily amount to an indefensible restrictive practice (chemical restraint)? Clearly, you will need to explore these issues with his parents tactfully to understand exactly what is going on with Alfred and his family.

References

(1) Hiscock H, Danchin MH, Efron D, Gulenc A, Hearps S, Freed GL, et al. Trends in paediatric practice in Australia: 2008 and 2013 national audits from the Australian Paediatric Research Network. *J Paediatr Child Health*. 2017;53(1):55–61.

(2) Ageranioti-Bélanger S, Brunet S, D'Anjou G, Tellier G, Boivin J, Gauthier M. Behaviour disorders in children with an intellectual disability. *Paediatr Child Health*. 2012;17(2):84–88.

(3) McDowell M. Neurodevelopmental and behavioural paediatrics. *J Paediatr Child Health*. 2015;51(1):113–117.

(4) Nicholls G, Bailey T, Grindle CF, Hastings RP. Challenging behaviour and its risk factors in children and young people in a special school setting: A four wave longitudinal study. *J Appl Res Intellect Disabil JARID*. 2023;36(2):366–373.

(5) World Health Organization. *International Classification of Functioning, Disability, and Health: Children & Youth Version: ICF-CY*. World Health Organization; 2007.

(6) United Nations. General Assembly, & Canada. Human Rights Directorate. *Convention on the rights of the child*. Human Rights Directorate; 1991.

(7) Executive Summary: Global report on children with developmental disabilities [Internet]. https://www.who.int/publications/i/item/9789240080539. Accessed 11 January, 2025.

(8) Weitzman C, Nadler C, Blum NJ, Augustyn M, Supporting Access for Everyone Consensus Panel. Health care for youth with neurodevelopmental disabilities: A consensus statement. *Pediatrics*. 2024;153(5):e2023063809.

(9) Anastasiou D, Kauffman JM. The social model of disability: Dichotomy between impairment and disability. *J Med Philos*. 2013;38(4):441–459.

(10) Macneil CA, Hasty MK, Conus P, Berk M. Is diagnosis enough to guide interventions in mental health? Using case formulation in clinical practice. *BMC Med*. 2012;10:111.

2

Causes of behaviour problems

The behaviour problem is not the problem. It's a symptom of the problem!

Consider a boy who has been diagnosed with Autism Spectrum Disorder (ASD) and who has aggressive behaviour at school. He hits other children. This generally follows his exclusion from games and being teased, in turn arising from his non-compliance with game rules. His school has not been able to prevent the teasing. His exclusion from games follows behaviours arising from his impaired social understanding and lack of empathy, a consequence of his ASD. His ASD is caused by a genetic aneuploidy known to be associated with ASD. A chain of causation has led to his challenging behaviour.

This chapter considers cause at all these levels. The chain of causation between explanatory factors and behaviour in some cases is direct, for example behaviours associated with a seizure disorder. In other cases, such as the example above, the pathway to causation occurs on multiple levels.

Child factors

Health

Behaviour may become problematic when children are unwell. This is particularly important for children not able to communicate about physical discomforts. Any of the following may underlie change in behaviour.

General health

1. Epileptic seizures
2. Injury—for example fractures, sprains, skin lesions
3. Infections—for example ears, respiratory, urinary

4. Immunological/inflammatory disorders

5. Dietary deficiencies

Pain and dysfunction

(For more information see (1).)

1. Ears, nose. and throat problems

2. Dental—for example caries, abscesses

3. Upper GI tract—gastroesophageal reflux, aspiration

4. Lower GI tract—constipation

5. Headaches

6. Any other causes of possible recurrent pain

> ## Practice tip: Think about health
>
> If there is sudden deterioration in behaviour of a non-verbal child, without obvious other cause, it is essential to search for a source of physical illness.

Lifestyle

1. Is the child tired? Sleep problems are common.

2. Is the child well nourished? (Look particularly in children with fussy eating/feeding problems).

3. Is the child active? Exercise and movement are central to function and development.

4. How does the child use screen technology (TV/Internet/games/social media)? In addition to being an adaptation to their predicament, use of social media can become an ongoing cause of problems (2). This includes lifestyle disruption (sleep/exercise/nutrition/hygiene), along with content-related behaviour disturbance.

Medical cause of disability

Medical assessment includes consideration of biological causation of developmental delays. A framework for thinking about medical aetiology includes:

◆ Genetic—present from conception

- Prenatal—intrauterine damage such as alcohol toxicity, failure to thrive, infections

- Perinatal—birth-related damage such as prematurity, infections, anoxia

- Postnatal—acquired damage such as brain injury. Included in this category would be the biological consequences of life experience as discussed below (e.g. neglect and abuse)

Specific conditions potentially provide specific information about child behaviour. An example is Prader–Willi syndrome. Another example is the specific patterns of neuropsychological impact following focal brain injury. For example, a child may have suffered a head injury with brain damage confined mainly to the frontal lobes. This child will be expected to display behaviour problems related to executive function deficits, such as impulsivity or apathy.

More generally, understanding of medical aetiology, known or presumed, informs understanding of a child's behaviour.

- **Influence on behaviour:** Common examples include irritability and fatigue associated with any painful condition and behaviour change before, during, and after a seizure.

- **Current capacity for choice:** To what extent does the child have the capacity to choose to manage situations differently? If they can change, to what extent is this sustainable?

- **Short term malleability:** To what extent is the problem amenable to therapeutic intervention, such as short-term therapy or behavioural strategy? Problems arising from significant neuropathology (e.g. severe intellectual disability) may be less malleable.

- **Natural history:** How might behaviours change over time with new learning and development, for example for a child who has not learned how to settle and make requests.

All these contributions to the understanding of behaviour are important and unique roles for the paediatrician. The contribution of specific conditions to understanding cause of behaviour problems is explored in Chapter 6.

Developmental competencies

This book considers children with developmental disabilities. By definition, they are not able to do all that typically developing children are able to do at the same chronological age. Rather than discuss what children are not able to do, the word 'competencies' is used to describe what a child is able to do, particularly with regards to their behaviour. Competencies represent the final common pathway for capacity (potential to learn), knowledge, and skills that are acquired developmentally.

When considering behaviour, it is important to know what a child is able to do as well as what they are not able to do. Families and schools manage children through expectations of what is reasonable and appropriate for children of different ages. An accurate understanding of a child's developmental competencies prevents misattribution, misinterpretation, and blame.

For children with developmental disabilities, both their rate of learning and current developmental capacities are likely to differ from default expectations. This difference may impact child behaviour in several ways. Some examples follow.

- The developmental problem may impact behaviour directly:
  - Behaviours that reflect impairments of emotional or impulse control
  - Behaviours associated with specific syndromes (e.g. the hyperphagia of Prader–Willi syndrome)
  - Behaviours that occur before, during, or after seizures
- The child is not able to do what is expected:
  - The child may become confused, scared, angry, frustrated in the situation, with behavioural consequences
  - Those with inaccurate expectations of a child's competence may perceive the child's behaviour as intentional (a behavioural problem) rather than arising due to the child's lack of capacity
- The child is not able to function effectively in the situation:
  - The non-verbal child cannot communicate their needs
  - The child with social problems has difficulty understanding the perspective and expectations of others
  - The child with a motor disorder may become fatigued and dysregulated

Practice tip: The child's experience

What is it like to be the child when demands and expectations are present? An appreciation of the individual child's competencies is the first step in 'seeing the world through the child's eyes'. What does the child understand? What are they able to do? What is their experience?

Measurement and communication of competencies

Methods for quantifying child abilities may include:

- Percentiles (place in the expected normal distribution for age)
- Standard scores (normalized by mean and standard deviation)
- Category results (e.g. average, below average)
- Descriptive results (e.g. mild, severe)

Common to all these is the challenge of mapping such information onto what the child can do in day-to-day life. For this purpose, a two-component structure is intuitive for parents and teachers alike:

1. **Age-equivalent, domain-specific function:** This characterizes a competency as approximately equivalent to a typically developing child of a particular age. An example is a 6-year-old child whose ability to understand and use language is at a 3-year-old age-equivalent level.

2. **Qualitative domain-specific differences:** This describes how the child's function differs from typically developing children of that age. An example is the child with a motor impairment, who may have additional struggles of fatigue with sustained effort, functional variability as they repeat the same task, and difficulty acquiring new skills. Another example is the child with intellectual disability who may have additional problems of attention and retention of information.

Intelligence

Intellectual capacities develop sequentially and may vary according to domains of information type, including language, social, visual, and spatial information.

Using the example of mathematics, intelligence enables the child to progress from rote counting to physical counting of objects to using numeric symbols, and on to increasing levels of conceptual abstraction (division, fractions, trigonometry, etc.).

Impairments of intelligence impact a child's capacity to comprehend information at an expected age level. In addition to children with Intellectual Disability (ID), there are three specific considerations:

- **Children with 'below average' intellectual capacity.** Their struggles are easily overlooked (3). Children with IQ 70 to IQ 85 are more common (~13.6%) than those whose IQ is less than 70 (~ 2.3%).
- **Children who are still too young for reliable IQ measurement** but are likely to have problems with cognition. This is termed 'global developmental delay' in children up to the age of 5 years in DSM5.

◆ **Diversity within cognitive profiles.** Intelligence is not a unitary attribute. There are multiple intelligences that can vary in the one individual. This may be strikingly evident in children with developmental disabilities. For example, children with autism may have savant skills as well as severely impaired social intelligence; children with Williams syndrome may have strong expressive language abilities but very weak visuospatial intelligence (see Chapter 6).

Problems of intelligence make it harder for children to find adaptive solutions to challenges they face. Behavioural consequences may arise from lack of understanding, along with their experience of confusion and emotions associated with this. In other cases, the chain of causation is not clear.

Language and communication

Language impairment is a fundamental and often overlooked cause of behaviour problems. Comprehension of language is necessary to understand what is being asked and expected of the child. Expressive skills enable children to say what they need, participate effectively in conversation, negotiate and resolve conflicts. Speech is a specific case of communicative competence. Problems of speech impact the sequencing, fluency and articulation of spoken language.

The predicament for children with language and communication problems is different from those with intellectual impairments. The language-impaired child has greater capacity to understand but cannot access or communicate that understanding through language. Children of ethnic minorities who use a different mother tongue face a similar challenge.

The child who does not understand in the first place, or who forgets what they have heard, may not follow instructions or may break rules. The child who has problems with expressive language and/or speech is likely to manage this struggle in accordance with their temperament. Resilient children may find another way to communicate. More sensitive children may withdraw from interaction, with selective mutism as an extreme example. Others may become frustrated and angry (with resulting behaviours) because their perspective is not recognized or understood.

Social competence

Social competence is arguably one of the most complex areas of developmental capacity. Social function combines several observable components.

Social intelligence: How well do children understand other people using information they receive (language, gesture, tone of voice, and other non-verbal information)? Social intelligence enables the child to use this information to understand others' thoughts, feelings, and motivations.

Social intelligence generally tracks overall intelligence. Problems may occur when social intelligence is less developed than general intelligence. This discrepancy is a central impairment for children with ASDs.

Social skills refer to acquired capacities to manage specific social challenges. This requires learning of social norms appropriate for age and context. Examples are participation in group activities for preschool children, and conflict resolution in older children.

Psychosocial development refers to the multifaceted processes by which social competency develops. How children understand themselves as part of their social system influences the behavioural choices they make. Social-emotional development is a related term that highlights the critical importance of the earliest stages of psychosocial development, a process that begins with responsive caregiving—and is an important predictor of life success. The ages and stages of typical psychosocial development are summarized in Table 2.1.

Further reading: The language of social skills

When considering age-appropriate social competency and related behaviour, a set of terms is commonly used.

- **Theory of mind** describes the child's capacity to understand the perspective of others—thoughts, feelings, and motivations.

- **Socio-emotional reciprocity** describes sequences of social interaction, for example imitation, turn-taking, affective matching. These behaviours may be readily observed in children before they learn to talk.

- **Pragmatics** of language refers to the use of language in a social context. This may include non-literal language, facial expression, and gesture use.

- **Empathy.** Like Theory of Mind, this describes the capacity to understand others. 'Empathy' is often used to characterize the emotional response of the individual to this understanding.

- **Sympathy** is the emotional response of the child when observing and understanding another's emotions, especially distress.

- **Social motivation** relates to a child's innate interest and desire for social connection.

A child's behaviour reflects their ability to understand the perspective of others, their situation-specific skills, and psychosocial developmental stage:

◆ The child with limited social intelligence may assume, for example, the other person believes, thinks, and feels the same way they do. Resulting behaviour may be misinterpreted as inappropriate, even wilful, rude, and disrespectful.

◆ The child with limited social skills may be unable to manage the resolution of different opinions and conflict. Typically, this occurs in association with problems of impulse control.

◆ The child with delayed psychosocial development manages social situations with developmental immaturity. A common example is the older child who

Table 2.1 Maladaptation to child disability and consequences for parenting

Family Issue	Possible Consequence for Parenting
Excessive guilt about the child's disability	Difficulty setting appropriate limits
Denial of disability	Unreasonable expectations on the child to perform normally
Chronic sadness	Lack of opportunity for family to have enjoyment
Unresolved denial	Never-ending quest to fix the child
Marked discrepancy between parents' attitude to the disability	Conflicting responses to child needs
Marked discrepancy between parents' attitude to behaviour problems (often worse with separated parents)	Ineffective and inconsistent behaviour management
Blame of one parent	Demoralized and disempowered parenting
Feeling overwhelmed by the child's disability	Disengagement from constructive management of behaviour
Shame	Inappropriate punishment of disabled child. Keeping the child away from social participation.
Survivor guilt in siblings	Siblings feel obliged to compensate in various ways

still behaves like a preschool aged child, with behaviours that are unco-operative and egocentric.

Executive functions, including attention and impulse control

Executive function refers to a set of abilities which collectively enable an individual to interpret, select, integrate, and remember incoming information, then consider, plan, and undertake action towards intended goals. The neuropsychology of these frontal lobe executive functions is complex, involving working memory, selective attention, and impulse control (see Further reading). Executive control systems consider purpose, generate plans, then undertake these plans with appropriate self-monitoring and self-control (4).

Further reading: Components of executive function

- **Attention control** is the capacity to allocate appropriate attentional focus to the task at hand.

- **Inhibitory control** is the capacity for age-appropriate consideration and choice in response to possible thoughts and actions.

- **Cognitive inhibition** is a specific case of inhibitory control, referring to the capacity to 'tune out' incoming stimuli that are irrelevant to the task at hand. In clinical terms this is the skill necessary to manage distractions.

- **Working memory** is the memory used during concentration, planning, and undertaking planned tasks. Working memory is biologically deter-mined and varies individually. Clinical assessment of working memory generally examines memory for different modalities (auditory and visual-spatial). Originally considered to be a fixed property of cognitive function, there is evidence that working memory can be modified with training (5).

- **Cognitive flexibility** enables us to adapt to changing demands. It re-quires ongoing monitoring and consideration of alternative strategies.

Observable behaviours arising from problems of executive function include many of the behaviours associated with Attention Deficit Hyperactivity Disorder (ADHD), for example impulsivity, hyperactivity, and inattention/distractibility. Such behaviours generally occur without the child's intention. The question 'why did you do that?' assumes that children have the capacity to intend, plan, remember, and control their behaviour. For children with impaired executive function, the valid answer to this question may be 'I don't know'.

Emotional regulation

Threat processing

Information coming into a child's nervous system is processed simultaneously along two pathways: one for interpretation and one for potential threat. Threat detection is a rapid, direct subcortical reaction to incoming information, without the luxury of preparatory or conceptual thinking. This system in the amygdala is closely integrated with hippocampal long-term memory.

Emotions arising in response to threat processing serve a motivational purpose (6). Threat processing systems operating in a healthy manner are able to generate emotions and behaviours appropriate for the situation at hand, such as a necessary 'fight, flight, or freeze' response.

Problems arise when threat detection and processing lead to the generation of emotions that are disproportionate to actual threat. This may occur, for example, when a child has experienced terror and hurt in the past, associated with loud voices. When they hear loud voices, they may respond as appropriate for a past, but not current threat.

Behaviours arising from problems of threat processing and labile affect can vary. Such variability can be observed, for example, comparing the child when healthy and feeling safe, to the same child when fatigued and emotionally vulnerable.

Biological systems of threat and affect control are vulnerable to life experience. When threat overwhelms a child's capacity to keep themselves safe ('toxic stress'), permanent changes may persist in biological systems of memory and emotional regulation (7). In this way, problems of the past exert continuing influence over the present.

Behaviour can be understood in the context of the child's emotional state at the time, a combination of type (e.g. anger) and intensity. Using a simple three-level metric (low, medium, high) of emotional intensity:

- **Low** levels do not substantially prevent a child's capacity to think with reasonable perspective and objectivity and behave with reasonable social maturity.

- **Medium** levels of emotional intensity make it more difficult for children to think and behave with objectivity and maturity. To do so may require substantial effort. There is a risk this effort will result in fatigue, with consequences for deterioration in self-control. In this state, small provocations carry a larger risk of triggering problematic behaviour.

- **High** levels of emotion lead to 'fight, flight, freeze' behaviours. They focus the central nervous system on the singular goal of survival. To achieve this, they take over control of thought as well as behaviour, so what children say when in this state may differ substantially from what they would say when calm.

Mood and affect

These terms are used somewhat variably in psychology. In this Guide, **affect** refers to **current** emotional state, such as happy, fearful, or angry. This varies in appropriateness and adaptation to circumstances.

Mood refers to persisting emotional states. Examples would be sustained depressed mood, or sustained periods of irritability, anger, excitement, or elation.

Both affect and mood may be emotional underpinnings of problem behaviour. A child with depressed mood is more likely to indulge in self-harm in response to loss or stress than a euthymic child. A child with angry affect is more likely to act aggressively if provoked than a child who is calm.

Academic learning

Problems of academic learning may arise for children because the curriculum may be inappropriate (too difficult or too easy), and/or the pedagogy is inappropriate (it does not match how the child learns). Child specific considerations include previous learning, intelligence, sensory function (vision, hearing), executive function, language, emotional regulation, and social competency.

Specific Learning Disorders (SLDs) (8) are defined by the domain of learning most affected (e.g. reading, mathematics, and written expression). SLD is common, affecting several in any classroom of typically developing children. Diagnostic criteria for SLD include response to intervention. Specifically, a child's rate of learning response is unexpectedly low for intervention considered appropriate and of sufficient duration.

Child behaviour problems potentially arise when curriculum and pedagogy are not appropriately adjusted and supported. Day after day, this causes persistent and recurrent stress. Over time, task avoidance may give way to resentment and anger, further impacting self-concept and school compliance.

Learning problems as a source of stress are relatively easy to identify during the primary school years, when children tend to have a single teacher and grade-structured classrooms. When learning problems present during the later years, however, they may be less obvious. As they are common, they should be considered in every case where a teenager's behaviour is not easy to understand.

Motor skills

As a domain of developmental competency, motor control is traditionally considered in three areas: oral motor (speech, feeding), fine motor (writing and other manipulative functions), and gross motor (general movement skills such as sport). A simple differentiation between upper extremity fine and gross is that fine motor control occurs beyond the wrist (finger dexterity). Oral motor is specific to speech and mouth function (chewing, swallowing).

Disorders of motor control have generally been categorized according to presence of neurological signs. When persistent signs are present, a child is likely to be diagnosed with cerebral palsy (gross motor) or dysarthria (oral motor). Motor control problems in the absence of 'hard' neurological signs fall in the category of dyspraxia, or Developmental Coordination Disorder. Motor control problems are common both as a primary issue (9), as well as comorbid with other problems (such as ADHD) (10).

The relationship between disorders of motor control and behaviour is similar to the situation with learning. If they are unable to meet expectations, stress accumulates, leading to inhibition, avoidance, or anger. With problems of motor coordination, children fatigue more quickly, leading to variability in capacity for behavioural self-control. Behaviour problems after school, for example when required to undertake homework or chores, may arise because children are just tired.

Temperament and personality

Temperament is the contribution of a child's innate make-up, separate to the consequences of childhood experience (11). Temperament describes properties of self-regulation and response to stimulation that are evident early in life. There is a substantial genetically transmitted contribution to temperament. Measurable dimensions of temperament include emotionality, adaptability and sociability. They generally remain a stable property of childhood personality structure over time (12).

Whilst temperament includes threat processing and affect control, it incorporates a larger set of traits (13). Temperament additionally refers to how children feel and respond to unfamiliar people and situations. Some children are sociable, some reserved. Some are energetic, outgoing, and reactive, whilst others may be quiet and inhibited.

Temperament influences children's responses to situations in a manner that is not readily amenable to change. For this reason, understanding and managing child behaviour involves understanding and working with each child's temperament.

Personality emerges as children with different temperaments experience life, interact, and learn. With time, patterns of response emerge and stabilize, becoming personality traits carried into adult life. Part of this process is the developmental acquisition of self-concept and self-esteem, as described below.

Strengths, interests, and resilience

Consideration of child competencies extends beyond evaluation of weaknesses and impairments. What child qualities exert a positive influence on behaviour?

Strengths refer to what a child may be innately good at. They set up a process whereby the child receives positive feedback when engaging in related activities. In this way, they influence self-concept and build self-esteem (see below). In general, they serve to positively motivate children. As they participate in activities that allow them to experience success and enjoy their strengths, children are more likely to manage their behaviour successfully.

Interests are also a source of positive motivation. Children with developmental disorders may have areas of relative strength, but absolute strengths may be difficult to identify. However, interests serve similar purposes with potentially greater utility. Interests enable a sense of purpose and pleasure. Participation in activities of interest builds identity within the group. These pathways collectively increase the probability of successfully adaptive behaviour.

Resilience refers to attributes that enable more successful management of stress. Children with greater resilience are less likely to behave in a problematic manner in stressful situations. Child resilience factors include (14–16):

◆ Calm, optimistic temperament

◆ Capacity to elicit positive responses from other people

◆ Positive friendships and social networks

◆ Higher intelligence, successful school experience

◆ Self-reliance, successful problem-solving skills

◆ Good self-esteem and self-concept

◆ Strengths, interests, including participation in associated activities

Impact of the child's past on current behaviour

When considering behaviour problems, understanding the child's past may provide valuable information that informs what is going on in the present.

Children internalize and encode what is experienced and learned over time, leading to neurobiological changes that persist. They become part of the child, long after the potentially harmful environments are no longer present, continuing to impact child behaviour, development, and mental health.

Attachment

Attachment is a complex developmental process that begins at birth (17) if not earlier. Donald Winnicott famously asserted (18) 'there's no such thing as a baby, only a baby–mother dyad'. Whilst attachment is a transactional process of early childhood, the consequences of disrupted attachment may persist throughout life.

Born fully dependent, a child experiences both their needs, and, simultaneously, the sensitivity and response of their caregiver. Children encode in memory this combination of need and caregiver response. Over time, repeated memories become a pattern that the child can use to predict future responses. A 'good enough' parent (19) is reliably, appropriately, and predictably responsive. In common language, the child is able to trust.

These integrated memories are encoded during what is considered to be a neurological 'critical' or 'sensitive' period (20) of neurological development, generally considered to be up to the age of 18 months. What is encoded during this time is likely to persist, even if a child's experiences subsequently change.

These early childhood experiences form foundational beliefs about the interpersonal world, the essential trustworthiness of those closest, on whom they depend. Expectations generated by the child (from early childhood experience) exert an ongoing influence over how they manage social relationships.

Disturbed early childhood attachment is likely to have lifelong consequences, with higher risk of mental health problems during teenage (21) and adult life. Various patterns of disturbed attachment have been described (e.g. insecure, avoidant, anxious, disinhibited, disorganized). More extensive reading is recommended if working with children whose background includes abuse/neglect (22).

Trauma and adverse life events

A central issue with early childhood trauma is the experience of overwhelming threat, fear, and pain by young children not able to defend themselves. Children who experience early childhood trauma may retain these learnings as a form of post-traumatic stress disorder (PTSD).

In later life, the clinical consequence is a misinterpretation of threat. The child may hear raised voices that elicit a memory of physical harm. A sudden gesture may trigger fear of being hit. Disinterest of others may trigger the threat of abandonment. The possibility that the child's behaviour may upset a significant figure in their life may terrify the individual because they expect disproportionate and harmful consequences.

Understanding what children have experienced in the past informs how current behaviour may be understood and managed. This involves understanding threat *as the child currently experiences it*. Understood in this way, it becomes clear when simple reassurance will be insufficient to help the child to feel safe.

Some common sources of adversity for children are (13):

- **Family dysfunction:** This includes interparental conflict and domestic violence, parental separation, and divorce. Family discord is strongly associated with children's behaviour problems. The effects of parental divorce are partly determined by the state of conflict following separation. Parental separation is also often followed by multiple losses such as the family home, school, and income security.

- **Parental mental disorder:** Children of parents with a mental illness are at lifelong risk of mental health and behavioural problems (23). Parent problems include severe personality disorders, alcoholism, and criminality. Parental mental illness leads to adversity and behaviour problems when the illness leads to poor parenting. This effect is largely mitigated if one parent has a healthy relationship with the child.

- **Neglect and abuse—current:** Children with disabilities are at increased risk of neglect and abuse (22). They are also at increased risk of sexual abuse, including from healthcare providers. This may be difficult to detect (24). The limited communication of many children with disabilities means they have impaired capacity to report what has happened to them. This makes them easy targets for potential abusers.

Paediatricians are familiar with the typical presentations of physical, emotional, and sexual abuse. However, some presentations are often overlooked in children with disabilities. In non-verbal children particularly, the occurrence of abuse should be suspected when there is an otherwise unexplained decline in function, or an unexpected change in behaviour, particularly when the child is in a situation (such as out-of-home care) where abuse is more likely. The decline in function may manifest in loss of independence skills, agitation, or depression.

◆ **Neglect and abuse—past:** Childhood abuse and neglect cause persisting brain changes with resulting long-term poor physical and mental health. Abuse has a negative effect on long-term cognitive development (25).

Goodman and Scott (14) describe four patterns of long-term emotional disturbance in children following abuse:

1. Emotional blunting and lack of social responsiveness.

2. Depressed affect with sad facial expressions, withdrawal, and aimless play.

3. Emotional lability, with sudden shifts from engagement and pleasure to withdrawal and anger; and

4. An angry emotional state with disorganized play and frequent outbursts in response to slight frustrations.

In adolescence, children who have suffered abuse have greatly increased rates of antisocial behaviour, and suicidal and self-harm behaviour. PTSD or other stress-related mental health problems are common. There is a high correlation between sexual abuse and the presence of Dissociative Disorder.

Practice tip: In for the long haul

The paediatrician is often asked to assist foster parents with the care of the previously abused child. A key message is that repair of the various biological and psychosocial sequelae takes many, not a few, years. It is a process, a journey, not a treatment event.

◆ **Poverty and adverse neighbourhoods:** This may be associated with problems in the community such as crime, violence, drug abuse, and low social cohesion. Socio-economic disadvantage is associated with behavioural problems in children. In children with mild intellectual disability and borderline intellectual function, disruptive behaviours are strongly associated with poverty (26). This effect appears to result from the disadvantaged neighbourhoods in which they live more than the poverty itself.

◆ **Racism and discrimination:** Children who grow up as victims of sustained discrimination, particularly racism, may suffer a wide range of adverse outcomes in physical, social, and psychological health. For more information a useful resource is this Harvard University 'useable knowledge' page.[1]

---

[1] How Racism Can Affect Child Development, November 2020; Accessed 12 November 2025, https://developingchild.harvard.edu/resources/infographics/racism-and-ecd/, 2025.

◆ **Poor schooling**: As discussed above, schools are a major social context for child development. Having a disability increases likelihood of bullying and other forms of trauma. Schools vary widely in their capacities to make accommodations and employ strategies necessary to manage learning, social, and behavioural needs.

◆ **Bullying, teasing, victimization**: Children who are perceived by their peers as odd or impaired, such as those with autism or intellectual disability, are more likely to be bullied. Victims of bullying during their schooling have increased rates of long-term mental health problems extending to young adulthood, including increased rates of depression, anxiety, and suicidal ideation (27). Many bullies are themselves victims of parental aggression and coercion.

◆ **War, famine, and displaced families**: For trauma of this magnitude, the child's capacity to cope will be intimately linked with the family's mental well-being. Family support will be the key intervention. Trauma is much greater if the child is separated from the family.

◆ **Pain, illness, and hospitalization**: These experiences heighten the child's dependency on attachment figures. Outcomes for children are worse when attachments are unreliable for, or unavailable to, the child.

Practice tip: Current trauma

Treatment of behaviour problems in situations of trauma is rarely successful while the trauma is ongoing. It is much more valuable for the paediatrician to support whatever action is necessary to end the current trauma.

Resilience to trauma

Resilience requires two fundamental safety properties of the child's world: these are access to key attachment figures, who are experienced as safe and nurturing, and protection from significant threats that arise from other people or the environment.

In addition, the following factors have been found to increase child resilience to trauma:

◆ A warm, close, and cohesive family.

◆ A supportive system for the family in the community, for example a church or extended family network.

◆ Outside support, for example a supportive school, especially with adult attachment figures who like and care for the child.

Self-concept and self esteem

Self-concept refers to beliefs about self that are acquired developmentally, shaped by the responses of significant others. This begins with parents, where concepts such as unconditional love, and 'good enough parenting' (28) frame what children learn about themselves.

As children grow and develop, the range of others who influence them becomes wider (see Table 2.1). The child assembles information to form beliefs about themselves on issues such as whether they are popular, smart, athletic, and/or attractive. These beliefs potentially exert increasing influence on behavioural choices made. An example is the confidence to try activities that are new.

Self-esteem arises from these self-concept beliefs according to how relevant or important that aspect of function is for the child. The child who values sporting competency is likely to have greater self-esteem if they are well coordinated and successful in sport.

Self-esteem may directly influence behaviour through its impact on motivation and capacity to engage with risk or uncertainty. As children gain autonomy, beliefs can become 'self-fulfilling prophecies'. For example, a child who believes they are 'bad' is more likely to make behavioural choices of that nature. If a particular behaviour (e.g. school avoidance) is strongly influenced by an underlying belief (e.g. I am bad at school) and associated emotions (e.g. shame), that behaviour is likely to be difficult to change whilst the belief and emotion persist.

Children with disabilities face additional threats to their self-esteem. A number of studies have shown lower self-esteem in children with developmental disabilities (e.g. (29)). Children with disabilities in regular schools are frequently subject to devaluation by other students, impairing their self-concept (30). This finding is not universal, however. Self-esteem of children with disabilities appears sensitive to the messages from others, just as with typically developing children.

Mental health disorders

A diagnosed mental disorder not only characterizes the nature of clinical problems for the child, it also provides information about expected natural history, possible causes, and treatment options. The challenges associated with specific mental health diagnoses are discussed further in Chapter 6.

The nature of the problem is likely to have a direct impact on behaviour—for example:

◆ The anxious child—behaviours of fear and avoidance

◆ The depressed child—behaviours that reflect reduced energy and motivation

◆ The child with a bipolar disorder—behaviours at the extremes of high and low arousal, behaviours that change markedly over time

◆ The child with a psychotic disorder—behaviours influenced by hallucinations, perceptual disturbance, or thought disorder

The child's world

The African proverb 'It takes a village to raise a child' remains true for children in the twenty-first century (31). There are many ways a child's world is relevant to the understanding and management of child behaviour. It may relate to how the child feels: do they feel safe, loved, visible, cared for? By contrast, is the world unsafe, such that the child is vigilant or frightened? Behaviour may reflect the world they live in. It may be the expression of what they observe and copy.

A child's world creates the context in which they grow and develop. With these contexts come expectations, such as helping around the house, or achieving curriculum. Children with developmental problems are likely to struggle with expectations if these are not adjusted to optimize the child's 'Goodness of Fit' (GOF). Successful GOF arises when expectations are fair, flexible, adaptive, reasonable, and sustainable for the individual child. It is a concept that applies at all clinical levels of child–environment interaction. Some examples are:

◆ **Immediate GOF:** The child's capacity to sustainably meet parent or school expectations (e.g. behaviour, social skills, curriculum requirements).

◆ **Context GOF:** The fit between the child's needs and the type of class they are in at school. For example, a child may function better at school when there is a low student-to-teacher ratio than in a class with 28 other students.

◆ **Values GOF:** Parents may have ambitions of academic performance that the child is unable to achieve or maintain.

When the 'fit' is poor, the child must adapt to the challenge of not being able to achieve, function, or behave as expected. Some may try to change and adapt, struggling when this is not sustainable. Some may distract or push back with their behaviour (e.g. aggression, defiance, being a 'clown'), whilst others may dissociate in some way, making themselves less 'visible'.

Family

The key social environment for children is the family. From general clinical practice, paediatricians develop an intuitive appreciation of the family's capacity to function appropriately and specifically act in the child's interest.

Many aspects of family dysfunction impact child's behaviour:

+ Modelled behaviours (e.g. losing temper, hitting)

+ Modelled capacities (e.g. how families regulate emotions, solve social problems)

+ Uncertain or inadequate behavioural boundaries

+ Poor lifestyle (sleep, exercise, food, media use) impacting the child's health, well-being, capacity to learn and self-control

+ Parentification, enmeshment, and other manifestations of disrupted family systems

These have consequences for the child:

+ Behaviours they consider normal and appropriate

+ Beliefs within the family, such as presumptions about authority figures (e.g. teachers), or instruction regarding how to manage conflict

+ Threat, the stress carried by children who don't feel safe at home

+ Worry that children carry about their parents and family

+ Beliefs the child may carry about themselves (e.g. inadequate, worthless) resulting from what they have been told at home

To build on this intuitive understanding, Skinner's Process Model (32) of family function provides a practical description.

Further reading: Skinner's Process Model

This model considers family from the perspective of function rather than structure. It includes seven key functions:

1. **Task accomplishment** refers to the capacity of the family to carry out basic tasks. These are conceived of as

   ○ **basic** tasks, such as providing food and shelter to the children;

   ○ **developmental** tasks, which refers to the capacity to carry out tasks which change as the child grows; and

○ **crisis** tasks, which refers to the ability to achieve essential goals in a crisis.

2. **Role performance** describes the extent to which each person is assigned different, appropriate roles within family life. This requires a willingness of family members to accept the assigned roles, along with capacity to actually undertake expected tasks.

3. **Effective communication** is necessary to ensure that roles and tasks are understood as intended. In addition, effective communication involves sharing of emotions as appropriate for situations.

4. **Emotional response** refers to the way individuals within the family respond emotionally to particular situations and stimuli.

5. **Affective involvement** refers to both the quality and degree to which family members express their interest in one another.

6. **Control** refers to the manner and degree to which family members influence (exert control over) each other.

7. **Values and norms** describe the beliefs and rules, both explicit and implicit, that direct and influence family behaviour. The impact of these values and norms is influenced also by the degree to which family values are shared by the surrounding culture.

Family systems

Skinner's model considers functions undertaken by the family. A different perspective to understanding families arises from systems theory (33). As a system, the family is more than a group of individuals. The system is the pattern of collective behaviour.

This system is defined by a boundary that differentiates the family from the outside. Within the boundary are matters of family privacy and roles taken by individuals. It is semipermeable in that other relatives and friends may be admitted within the boundary for a limited purpose or time. With time, individual family members move beyond the family boundary as they form their own links with others.

A family has subsystems: parents are one subsystem, the siblings another, and grandparents may be another. These subsystems also have their own semipermeable boundaries which evolve over time. Patterns of system or subsystem interactions have an impact on individual children. The behaviour of an individual child may arise from their involvement in these system patterns.

The child with disability in the family

The presence of a child with a disability within the family presents a challenge. For parents, there may be excess focus on the disabled child, to the neglect of the needs of other family members (parents and siblings). The child with disability may be a source of shame. The child may be rejected to some extent, particularly if their behaviours are interpreted as intentionally disruptive.

The challenge for siblings is also significant. They may behave with embarrassment, avoidance, or hostility. They may suffer resentment, anger, survivor guilt, and/or fear of responsibility for their sibling now and into the future.

The healthiest family adaptation is where the child with the disability is seen as equally important as other family members, not more important nor less important.

A healthy family adaptation to the disabled child will set the foundation for family care in the future. The parents will reach the age where they are unable to care for their disabled offspring. This duty may then devolve to the non-disabled siblings, whose willingness to take on this role is strongly influenced by the family's response to the disabled child when all the children are young.

Bereavement

Every parent wants to have a healthy child. When a family has a child with a disability, the family experiences the loss of the wished-for child. Grief associated with loss is processed as bereavement, and resolution of the family's bereavement has a significant impact on the behaviour of the child with a disability.

Kubler-Ross' stages of grief are clinically useful to understand what the families may be experiencing (34). These stages are denial, anger, bargaining, depression, and acceptance. Working through these stages is not necessarily a journey through definable sequential phases. When children have ongoing disability, even healthy, adaptive bereavement is likely to be variable, with chronic recurrent sorrow (35) potentially triggered by particular experiences or transitions. Each failure of the child with a disability to meet milestones which matter to the family is a source of further bereavement.

Practice tip: Sorrow is recurrent

There are times when parents are confronted with their disabled child's differences. At these times, the child's struggle in comparison with other children is unavoidably evident. Examples include commencing school, transition to high school, and preparing for life after school. As a clinician, be mindful of the recurrent grief that arises on these occasions.

The journey of bereavement can go astray in a more sustained manner. Bonnano (36) describes four different possible trajectories bereavement may take:

◆ **Resilience**—sustained functional strength throughout.

◆ **Recovery**—initial grief and dysfunction, then getting back on a healthy track.

◆ **Chronic dysfunction**—an unresolving cycle of function alternating with grief and impaired capacity to manage.

◆ **Delayed grief or trauma**—initial resilience (often with denial), followed by deterioration at an unexpected time.

Successful bereavement, acceptance, and adaptation is associated with the ability to attribute some positive meaning to loss. This was the teaching of Victor Frankel, a psychiatrist who survived Auschwitz (Frankel, *Man's search for meaning*. Beacon Press; 1946). For example, parents whose child has died from a rare disease may establish a support group for other parents or a foundation for research into the disease. This enables the parents to feel that the loss of their child has meant that other affected families will not have to suffer as much.

Patterns of family dysfunction

Table 2.1 describes some of the common patterns of family dysfunction and the behavioural consequences often observed in the child with disability.

Separated parents

With the high prevalence of parental separation, most paediatricians will have considerable experience working with children who live across different households. This can be a difficult, often irresolvable challenge. When parents are unable to work together for the benefit of their child in the relationship, they are even less likely to do so after separation. These challenges are greater when children have disabilities.

Parental alienation

A fundamental principle of family law is that children have the right to a meaningful relationship with each parent. Parental alienation is a problematic form of conflict between separated parents (37) that violates this principle. The term has been used to describe a process in which one parent actively undermines a child's relationship with the other parent (38) and may be considered a form of child abuse (39). A child's developmental needs can be used by parents to exaggerate differences between parenting beliefs and styles, sometimes to the point where it meets criteria for parental alienation. Alienation behaviours range from overt criticism to subtle forms of undermining masquerading as concern for the other parent.

The initial challenge for paediatric care is to be aware of parental alienation and the effects on the child. The impact of alienation on child behaviour varies considerably, depending particularly on the child's age in addition to other factors. Behaviour may be restricted to one household. It may include withdrawal, depression, oppositionality, and aggression. The impact on school function is often significant. When present, it becomes particularly important for the paediatrician to maintain the distance and objectivity necessary to avoid collusion with either parent. For specific cases, the advice of professional colleagues may be helpful.

School

For most children, school is their second most significant social environment. When the child has a disability, a crucial factor will be the flexibility the school has in adapting to the child's differences from the school 'norm'. When determining properties of the school, and how these may impact on child behaviour, the following considerations can be understood in terms of fit between child capacity and school circumstance:

1. **Curriculum**: Is the child able to meet curriculum expectations reliably and sustainably?

2. **Teacher**: Children thrive with teachers who are clear, consistent, firm, fair, and reliable. In high school particularly, teenagers work better with teachers they like, and who understand and like them in return.

3. **Behaviour strategy**: What happens when the child breaks the rules? Is the response appropriate, proportionate, fair, consistent, constructive?

4. **Bullying**: How safe is the school for this child? What is their attitude to bullying, and how do they manage it? Is there a bullying culture within the school's administration and teaching staff? How do they manage the individual child or group who bullies, and how do they manage the child who is bullied?

5. **Communication**: If a child has special needs, to what extent is that information communicated between staff, and with peers as appropriate? How well does the school communicate with parents and children themselves?

6. **Class Structure**: Is the child in a class type appropriate for his support needs? For example, a child with limited capacity to socialize may behave better in a class with fewer students.

7. **School culture**. At a whole school level, what are the priorities and constraints?

- ○ **Children:** What aspects of child development are important for that school? What is celebrated on the walls, in assembly meetings? Is it academic, social, and sporting achievement, or is it the individual value and worth of each child.

- ○ **Family and community:** To what extent does the school welcome the involvement of family and participate in the local community?

- ○ **Administration:** How do the senior administration manage the school staff? Is the culture supportive, respecting contribution, effort, innovation? Is the culture bureaucratic, indifferent, or punishing towards staff?

- ○ **Beliefs and values:** How does the school determine values, particularly those that guide child behavioural expectations? In religious schools, for example, expectations may be powerfully influenced by religious doctrines.

- ○ **Stress:** What current issues may be a stress for the school (e.g. staff shortages).

When behaviour problems occur in one environment but not another

A common challenge managing behaviour is that it may vary considerably across environments. Examples include the child who behaves acceptably at school but not at home. Another is the child living across households, with different behaviours in each. There are several possible explanations for this.

- ◆ **Behavioural barometer:** A child's goodness-of-fit experience may differ markedly across environments. Home may be adaptive and supportive, for example, whilst school is poorly aligned to the child's needs, especially if the child has significant disability. In this situation, the child's response is a form of 'behavioural barometer' that provides information about the environment within which behaviour occurs.

- ◆ **The stress of maintaining control:** A different situation occurs when children experience poor fit in one environment, however they have the capacity to control their frustration, distress, and behaviour. It may be important for the child, for example, to manage what other children think of them, or avoid getting into trouble at school. This stress accumulated in the effort to achieve this is brought home, where its release results in problematic behaviour. In contrast to the 'behavioural barometer', this 'good/bad' pattern arises when stress in one environment is released in another, where the child feels safe to do so.

The child's community and social ecology

Beyond the immediate or direct level of social context (family, school, friends, community), there are several additional, indirect levels of social ecology that influence child behaviour, particularly how it is understood and managed. Bronfenbrenner's ecological systems (40) approach is a useful way to think about this.

The community and ecology relevant to a child's behaviour includes the family's cultural and religious environment. For teenagers, this includes the beliefs and values held by their network of friends.

Social media is a growing area of influence for many aspects of child development, including beliefs, values, behaviours, and mental health (41). Children with developmental disorders are potentially more vulnerable to the influence of social media, particularly cyber-bullying (42). Another danger of social media is identification with unhealthy groups, for example websites that encourage anorexic behaviour. The harmful messages of social media may bypass the family's efforts to support and protect children. This vulnerability is more likely to be a problem when families are dysfunctional.

Excessive use by children of smartphones and computers is a global concern, and children with disabilities—especially ASD—may be especially susceptible to the allure of videogames and social media content. Children and adolescents may become more socially isolated and withdrawn, with downstream effects on sleep, school performance, friendships, and family conflict.

Further reading: Bronfenbrenner's ecological systems

- The **Microsystem** is the level of direct contact (family, school, community, etc.).

- The **Mesosystem** is the system that manages how these different microsystems communicate and collaborate. A common example is how well schools and families work together.

- The **Exosystem** is the social structures, organizations, and service systems (culture, values) that influence the meso- and microsystems. An example may be government policy, or religious beliefs that influence school behaviour management.

- The **Macrosystem** refers to society as a whole, including socio-economic, racial, and cultural considerations.

◆ Bronfenbrenner's final layer is time—the **Chronosystem**. This could be considered intrinsic to any child developmental perspective on behaviour.

Learned behaviour

Learned behaviours are included in this section of the child's world because learned behaviours can be understood as the external world internalized by the child. Learned behaviours derive from experience but persist after that experience has ceased. Some learned behaviours become embedded, difficult to alter with standard behaviour management. Others are more malleable.

Paediatricians benefit from an understanding of basic learning theory for several reasons:

◆ To understand aspects of a child's behaviour that are strongly determined through behavioural learning.

◆ To design and undertake behaviourally based interventions themselves.

◆ To understand and to follow psychological reports and therapeutic strategies provided to their patients. This is important when guiding parents, and determining co-management contributions such as use of medication.

Further reading: Behavioural learning theory

Classical conditioning refers to the process whereby a reflex or reactive behaviour becomes associated with a new stimulus that does not originally provoke the behaviour. An example would be where a child has been injured in a crash involving the car in which the child was travelling and a bus. Afterwards, the child has a reflex fear reaction whenever he sees a bus.

Operant conditioning refers to learning which results from the child's actions, rather than reflex responses. If the child's action results in a reward or pleasant consequences, the child tends to repeat it. If it results in an unpleasant experience, the behaviour diminishes.

Star charts and similar strategies are based on operant conditioning. Behaviour modification in children with developmental disabilities commonly comprises ignoring undesirable behaviours and rewarding desirable ones.

Reinforcement. Reinforcement serves to increase a particular behaviour. In the most part, this is positive reinforcement, or reward for behaviour. Skinner described patterns of reinforcement depending on the relationship between behaviour and reward over time.

- **Continuous** reinforcement, where the reward is given every time, produces the quickest learning, but not necessarily the most persistent learning. It can also diminish quickly when the reward is no longer present.

- **Intermittent** (partial) reinforcement produces learning which may occur more slowly but lasts longer after the reward is stopped.

Negative reinforcement refers to the removal of an unpleasant stimulus when the desired behaviour is undertaken. An example is the beeping noise in a car that stops when a seat belt is plugged in.

Punishment. In contrast to reinforcement, punishment serves to decrease behaviour. It links a consequence to behaviour that the child does not like. For children with developmental disorders, punishment may be inappropriate, ineffective, and potentially abusive if the child is not able to understand what is needed, or able to readily and sustainably behave in the expected manner. Reinforcement, particularly positive, is considered more effective than punishment for sustained behaviour change.

Further reading: Social learning theory

Social learning theory examines how behaviours can be learned by observing and imitating others. For children, it characterizes the effect of behaviours observed by the child, for example, in the family home. The pioneer of this work was Bandura (43). Social learning has been described within two processes (44).

- **Observational learning** is the process whereby children learn from imitating the actions of others. Identification is learning by copying the general style of others, particularly important people in the child's life.

- **Contextual control analysis** describes the observation that the strength of reinforcement depends on its context. For example, if a child is given an edible treat as a reward, then it will be most influential if that treat is seldom available to the child. It might also be more potent if the child has not recently been eating.

Resilient and supportive environments

Aspects of the child's environment support a child's positive development and mental health and lower the risk of problem behaviour. Identifying and enhancing these can be useful in the management of difficult behaviour. An example is enabling a child to spend more time with a relative (e.g. grandparent) who accepts the child unconditionally, and with whom the child can relax and have fun.

Environment level resilience factors identified in research include:

- Supportive adults (parents, teachers) who understand and unconditionally accept the child
- Capacity and willingness to adapt to the child's individual needs
- Economic sufficiency and stability
- Loving, reasonable, fair, and predictable environments
- Capacity for calm and effective problem-solving
- Stability over time
- Access to opportunities to develop interests and strengths
- Adults who set consistent limits

Practice tip: Start with the strengths

When the child's world seems very dysfunctional, so that it appears hard to find a way to intervene positively, it's a good idea to search for any point of strength in the child's world and try to support that. It could be someone outside the immediate family, for example a more distant relative, a school teacher, a football coach, etc.

Chapter summary

Problem behaviour arises as the final common pathway for multiple potential causes, with contributing factors falling across the biological-psychological-social continuum.

Child factors relevant to causes of behaviour problems include:

◆ Current health issues

◆ Medical conditions, including brain pathology and inherited vulnerability to mental disorders

◆ Current developmental competencies: what they are able to do, what they find difficult, how well they are able to meet expectations

◆ Temperament/personality

◆ The child's past, how this has been internalized and influences the present

◆ Strengths and other child-specific resilience factors

Factors in the child's environment that influence child behaviour include:

◆ Current safety

◆ Family

◆ School

◆ Community

◆ Behaviour that is observed and copied by the child

◆ Supportive and resilient environments

Appendix 2.1—Development of self-concept: Ages and stages

Children learn about themselves through their interactions with the world in which they live. This occurs in a developmental sequence with regards to who has the greatest influence on child self-concept, and the flexibility/permanence of resulting beliefs (45).

Preschool: In the preschool years, self-concept mainly derives from parents, siblings, close family, and friends. The world of children is small, so they are not in a position to put this information in a larger context.

Primary school age: As children progress through primary school, they are likely to know what their parents believe, becoming less reliant on parental opinion. Instead, they are more influenced by authority figures (e.g. teachers) and the opinions of their peers. If what they are told is not in line with what they experience, however, they are more likely to believe what they experience.

Early adolescence. This is a time of change with biological urges associated with puberty. Psychologically, beliefs become more personal, less amenable particularly to parental opinion. It is the beginning of a transition process towards independence, not only in life but also in self-concept.

Late adolescence: The developmental drivers of adolescence work towards increasing independence. As a result, the sources of information of greatest relevance are those with whom the youth most strongly identifies. This includes their peer group, but also includes teachers with whom they feel a sense of affinity (being understood and liked). Information on social media is an increasingly important consideration. Such information tends to be optimized (people share what is their very best), increasing the comparison discrepancy when youth self-reflect against these measures.

Appendix 2.2—Ages and stages of social development

How a child 'fits in' to the social world is something they learn in social development. A useful framework for this is the work of Erik Erikson (46), which can be interpreted from the perspective of normal child behavioural development within a social context.

Up to 18 months: Trust vs Mistrust. The child's psychosocial focus is on the predictability of the care they receive. This results in secure attachment as described above, simply understood as capacity to trust those on whom they depend. During this time, they begin to build a sense of independent identity within the safety of trustworthy relationships.

18 months to 3 years: Autonomy vs Shame/Doubt. From a secure base of trust, the child builds autonomy, for example with walking and talking. Their social perspective is necessarily egocentric, not yet able to fully understand themselves in the context of family and other social groupings. As the child learns to control themselves, they may object to the perception that others are attempting to control them.

3 to 5 years: Initiative vs Guilt. Using the skills acquired, children interact and learn. In doing so, they are open to the opinions of others. If they feel confident, they try new things. If they feel inadequate or guilty, they may resist. They are finding their place, revising their identity, in a larger social world.

5 to 12 years: Industry vs Inferiority. In primary school (latency) years, this process of learning and developing continues. From a social perspective, children learn about themselves in the context of peers and teachers as well as family. These beliefs inform their capacity to take risks, manage mistakes, to cooperate, to compromise, and other social behaviours related to ongoing learning and function. It is an important time for the construction of identity (see below).

12 to 18 years: Identity vs Confusion. In adolescence, the journey of personal identity within the social world continues, extending to becoming an independent individual. Identity is necessarily differentiated from what family in particular expects. Instead, identity with respect to peer groups is likely to take precedence. Differentiation does not mean division and separation, however. Successful differentiation enables the young adult to remain in relationship (family, friends), but to do so confidently as themselves.

Appendix 2.3—Clinical cases

These cases continue from those presented in Chapter 1.

Case 1. Jack

You know Jack's behaviour is harmful to himself and to others, so it is appropriate for paediatric care. This extends beyond the use of ADHD medication. To understand what may work, it is first necessary to understand the set of contributing causes. This assessment of causes should serve as the basis of a management plan.

Discussion

What else do you need to know about Jack?

Jack had a multidisciplinary assessment as part of his Foetal Alcohol Spectrum Disorder (FASD) diagnosis. In addition to the summary report, it may be useful to obtain details of his cognitive profile, language, and executive function.

Jack's forgetfulness and impulsivity may contribute to his problem behaviour despite ongoing stimulant therapy. It is likely that he experiences frustration and failure in many areas of his life (e.g. learning, friendships), causing problematic behavioural responses to these challenges. He may have trouble using language to understand and negotiate behavioural situations. His capacity to understand expected social boundaries may be below age and grade expectations. From his early childhood experience he may have unresolved attachment issues and residual problems with trust.

What else do you need to know about Jack's family?

We need to know about Jack's life before the foster placement. Was there other drug use or a history of neglect or abuse? Childhood trauma may raise the possibility of attachment disorder and PTSD in addition to FASD.

We need to understand how his family makes sense of Jack's behaviour currently, looking for fairness, consistency, and clarity in their behaviour management. A common misconception carried by parents who foster and adopt children from abuse backgrounds is a belief that consistent love and care will 'overcome' the consequences of early childhood adversity. Jack's family may be struggling with the fact that his behaviour is not settling down, that he does not appear to trust them, to understand he is 'safe'. The family may need information and support to understand the consequences of early childhood abuse and neglect even beyond the consequences of FASD and ADHD.

Finally, we need to understand the general well-being of the family. Managing a child like Jack is a consistent source of stress, fatigue, and possible demoralization. Ongoing strength, resilience, and empowerment for the family is the foundation of Jack's ongoing success.

What else do you need to know about Jack's school?

We need to know details of what he does, where, how often, and how long the behaviour lasts. With regards to the context, this includes the situational triggers, what seems to perpetuate the behaviour, and what works to settle it down.

The school may assert Jack has an individualized educational curriculum and imply that his learning needs are appropriately met, which may or may not be true. We may need to understand how they have adapted the curriculum, ensuring what is provided is within his capacity to achieve and sustain success.

Other information may be relevant, such as his peer relationships, bullying, strategies that work to prevent behavioural episodes, what Jack likes and is good at, and whatever else helps you understand the school experience from Jack's point of view.

Case 2. Jade

Jade is a 14-year-old girl in her second year of high school. She has a diagnosis of mild, high function ASD made four years earlier. Her behaviour has been worsening across the last 12 months, with angry non-compliant behaviour at home, and school avoidance. Jade's behaviour is harmful to herself (e.g. school avoidance consequences) and others (e.g. hitting her younger brother and verbally demeaning him). She has little insight into how others may see her or be impacted by her behaviour, with strongly argued beliefs regarding how fault lies with others (teachers, peers, and family members).

Discussion

What might be contributing to the challenging behaviour, both increasing and decreasing it?

If Jade is to return to school, she needs to feel safe and supported in meeting social and academic challenges. Jade may have an underlying problem with executive function or a Specific Learning Disability. Socially, Jade may just feel different, lonely, and isolated, or perhaps she is being ostracized or bullied.

As Jade is age 14, it is important for you to have some understanding of her personal life. Of potential relevance are use of drugs (e.g. marijuana), gender identity, what she spends time doing on social media, and so on.

Jade's parents may feel blamed and responsible for their daughter's behaviour. Their behaviour management strategies may be inconsistent and ineffective.

Case 3. Alfred

Alfred is a 6-year-old boy with Down syndrome and moderate Intellectual Disability (ID). Since your earlier visit (Chapter 1), Alfred's parents have separated and he is living with his mother. Satisfied that there was no physical abuse of Alfred, you made a referral to a child and family therapist. The therapist has provided support to Alfred's mother while helping Alfred's father in understanding Alfred's limitations. Although they continue to have disagreements about Alfred, their overt conflict has improved. Consequently, his disruptive and aggressive behaviours have decreased substantially both in school and at home.

Recent psychological assessment shows that Alfred's cognitive and language abilities are at around 2.5 years age equivalent. The psychologist noted his very short attention span and a high degree of impulsivity.

On this follow-up visit, his mother reports that Alfred's behaviour has changed over the last few weeks. He is becoming uncharacteristically tearful, angry, and uncooperative, and during these episodes he sometimes hits his face and head. Other changes include a reduction in appetite and greater sleep disruption. His behaviour does not indicate a focus for pain and he has been in good general health. There have been no changes with regard to visitation or family home environment. Alfred is a difficult child to examine. He is resistant to examination of his mouth and ears.

Discussion

What particular health issues are important to consider in a child with Down syndrome that may impact Alfred's behaviour?

It is important to consider health issues in a child with disabilities when there is evidence of deteriorating behaviour. In children with Down syndrome, you should consider middle ear disease and hypothyroidism, in addition to the other 'usual suspects' (dental problems, gastroesophageal reflux, and constipation). At the same time, inquire about changes in the child's life at home or at school that might be causal.

In this case, further evaluation of potential health problems led to diagnosis of severe dental caries and periapical abscess. His behaviour improved after surgical treatment.

How do the findings from the psychological assessment help you in understanding Alfred's behaviour?

We are told that Alfred's psychological assessment showed severe cognitive and language impairment. All too often, valuable findings from skilled assessments by psychologists, speech-language pathologists, and other professionals are not communicated effectively to families and caregivers. You can use the assessment findings as an opportunity to provide psychoeducation, emphasizing to them that his understanding is like that of a 2-year-old child. You may suggest very simple instructions and visual supports to help Alfred with transitions.

References

(1) Street K. Pain in children with severe intellectual disability. 2015.

(2) Zebracki K. The good, the bad, and social media in adolescents with disability. *Dev Med Child Neurol.* 2019;61(8):856.

(3) Emerson E, Einfeld S, Stancliffe RJ. The mental health of young children with intellectual disabilities or borderline intellectual functioning. *Soc Psychiatry Psychiatr Epidemiol.* 2010;45(5):579–587.

(4) Diamond A. Executive functions. *Annu Rev Psychol.* 2013;64(1):135–168.

(5) Fitamen C, Blaye A, Camos V. Five-year-old children's working memory can be improved when children act on a transparent goal cue. *Sci Rep.* 2019;9(1):15342.

(6) Barrett LF, Lewis M, Haviland-Jones JM, eds. *Handbook of Emotions.* 4th ed. The Guilford Press; 2016.

(7) Cooke EM, Connolly EJ, Boisvert DL, Hayes BE. A systematic review of the biological correlates and consequences of childhood maltreatment and adverse childhood experiences. *Trauma Violence Abuse*. 2023;24(1):156–173.

(8) McDowell M. Specific learning disability. *J Paediatr Child Health*. 2018;54(10):1077–1083.

(9) Shaywitz SE, Shaywitz JE, Shaywitz BA. Dyslexia in the 21st century. *Curr Opin Psychiatry*. 2021 Mar 1;34(2):80–86. doi:10.1097/YCO.0000000000000670. PMID: 33278155.

(10) Goulardins JB, Marques JCB, De Oliveira JA. Attention deficit hyperactivity disorder and motor impairment. *Percept Mot Skills*. 2017;124(2):425–440.

(11) Zwir I, Arnedo J, Del-Val C, Pulkki-Råback L, Konte B, Yang SS, et al. Uncovering the complex genetics of human temperament. *Mol Psychiatry*. 2020;25(10):2275–2294.

(12) Kopala-Sibley DC, Olino T, Durbin E, Dyson MW, Klein DN. The stability of temperament from early childhood to early adolescence: A multi-method, multi-informant examination. *Eur J Personal*. 2018;32(2):128–145.

(13) Thapar A, Pine DS, Leckman JF, Scott S, Snowling MJ, Taylor EA, eds. *Rutter's Child and Adolescent Psychiatry*. 6th ed. Wiley-Blackwell; 2015.

(14) Goodman R, Scott S. *Child and Adolescent Psychiatry*. 3rd ed. Wiley-Blackwell; 2012.

(15) Masten AS, Best KM, Garmezy N. Resilience and development: Contributions from the study of children who overcome adversity. *Dev Psychopathol*. 1990;2(4):425–444.

(16) Werner EE. Resilient children. *Young Child*. 1984;40:68–72.

(17) Rutter M. Clinical implications of attachment concepts: Retrospect and prospect. *J Child Psychol Psychiatry*. 1995;36(4):549–571.

(18) Winnicott DW. The theory of the parent–infant relationship. *Int J Psychoanal*. 1960;41:585–595.

(19) Winnicott DW. Transitional objects and transitional phenomena; a study of the first not-me possession. *Int J Psychoanal*. 1953;34(2):89–97.

(20) Opendak M, Sullivan RM. Unique neurobiology during the sensitive period for attachment produces distinctive infant trauma processing. *Eur J Psychotraumatology*. 2016;7:31276.

(21) Seim AR, Jozefiak T, Wichstrøm L, Lydersen S, Kayed NS. Self-esteem in adolescents with reactive attachment disorder or disinhibited social engagement disorder. *Child Abuse Negl*. 2021;118:105141.

(22) Legano LA, Desch LW, Messner SA, Idzerda S, Flaherty EG, Council on Child Abuse and Neglect, et al. Maltreatment of children with disabilities. *Pediatrics*. 2021;147(5):e2021050920.

(23) Brummelhuis IAM, Kop WJ, Videler AC. Psychological and physical wellbeing in adults who grew up with a mentally ill parent: A systematic mixed-studies review. *Gen Hosp Psychiatry*. 2022;79:162–176.

(24) Kvam MH. Is sexual abuse of children with disabilities disclosed? A retrospective analysis of child disability and the likelihood of sexual abuse among those attending Norwegian hospitals. *Child Abuse Negl*. 2000;24(8):1073–1084.

(25) Shonkoff JP, Garner AS, Committee on Psychosocial Aspects of Child and Family Health, Committee on Early Childhood, Adoption, and Dependent Care, Section on

Developmental and Behavioral Pediatrics. The lifelong effects of early childhood adversity and toxic stress. *Pediatrics*. 2012;129(1):e232–246.

(26) Emerson E, Einfeld S. Emotional and behavioural difficulties in young children with and without developmental delay: A bi-national perspective. *J Child Psychol Psychiatry*. 2010;51(5):583–593.

(27) Wolke D, Lereya ST. Long-term effects of bullying. *Arch Dis Child*. 2015;100(9):879–885.

(28) Winnicott DW. *The Child, the Family, and the Outside World*. Penguin Books; 1964.

(29) Zeleke S. Self-concepts of students with learning disabilities and their normally achieving peers: A review. *Eur J Spec Needs Educ*. 2004;19(2):145–170.

(30) Gurney PW. *Self-Esteem in Children with Special Educational Needs*. Routledge; 2018.

(31) Reupert A, Straussner SL, Weimand B, Maybery D. It takes a village to raise a child: Understanding and expanding the concept of the 'village'. *Front Public Health*. 2022;10:756066.

(32) Skinner H, Steinhauer P, Sitarenios G. Family Assessment Measure (FAM) and process model of family functioning. *J Fam Ther*. 2000;22(2):190–210.

(33) Papero DV. *Bowen Family Systems Theory*. 1st ed. Pearson; 1990.

(34) Tyrrell P, Harberger S, Schoo C, Siddiqui W. Kubler-Ross Stages of Dying and Subsequent Models of Grief. In: *StatPearls* [Internet]. StatPearls Publishing; 2022. http://www.ncbi.nlm.nih.gov/books/NBK507885/

(35) Hobdell EF, Deatrick JA. Chronic sorrow: A content analysis of parental differences. *J Genet Couns*. 1996;5(2):57–68.

(36) Bonanno GA. Loss, trauma, and human resilience: Have we underestimated the human capacity to thrive after extremely aversive events? *Am Psychol*. 2004;59(1):20–28.

(37) Bernet W, Greenhill LL. The five-factor model for the diagnosis of parental alienation. *J Am Acad Child Adolesc Psychiatry*. 2022;61(5):591–594.

(38) Harman JJ, Warshak RA, Lorandos D, Florian MJ. Developmental psychology and the scientific status of parental alienation. *Dev Psychol*. 2022;58(10):1887–1911.

(39) Isailă OM, Hostiuc S. Medical-legal and psychosocial considerations on parental alienation as a form of child abuse: A brief review. *Healthc Basel Switz*. 2022;10(6):1134.

(40) Bronfenbrenner U. *The Ecology of Human Development: Experiments by Nature and Design*. Harvard University Press; 1979.

(41) Bozzola E, Spina G, Agostiniani R, Barni S, Russo R, Scarpato E, et al. The use of social media in children and adolescents: Scoping review on the potential risks. *Int J Environ Res Public Health*. 2022;19(16):9960.

(42) Touloupis T, Athanasiades C. Cyberbullying and empathy among elementary school students: Do special educational needs make a difference? *Scand J Psychol*. 2022;63(6):609–623.

(43) Bandura A. *Social Learning Theory*. 1st ed. Prentice-Hall; 1976.

(44) Birch A, Malim T. *Introductory Psychology*. Bloomsbury Publishing; 2017.

(45) Harter S, Bukowski WM. *The Construction of the Self: Developmental and Sociocultural Foundations*. 2nd ed. The Guilford Press; 2015.

(46) Erikson EH. *Childhood and Society*. W W Norton & Co; 1950.

3

Assessment

Behaviour is measurable. So measure it!

Standard medical assessment attempts to answer two central questions:

1. What is the nature of the presenting problem (history over time, extent, and impact on the child)?

2. What is (are) the cause(s) of this problem? What further assessment or investigation needs to be done to clarify this?

Assessment to understand behaviour problems is no different. Chapter 1 discussed behaviour as a problem amenable to medical thinking. Chapter 2 discussed possible causes of behaviour problems.

This chapter addresses practical challenges and strategies of assessment. In addition to assessment of the child, this extends to the child's family, school, and community, thereby covering the relevant bio-psycho-social range of possible contributing factors.

As noted earlier, it is assumed the paediatrician is familiar with general medical and developmental assessment. Strategies discussed below are specific to evaluation of behaviour and possible causes.

If a child has multiple behaviour problems, each of which is individual in nature or type, each behaviour type may require both independent understanding (diagnostic formulation, Chapter 4) and management strategy (Chapter 5) as well as assessment.

Prior to attendance, or in the waiting room

Background information

How information is collected depends on practice style (e.g. paper based, Internet based), and the amount of information you have available prior to the consultation visit.

- If it is known beforehand that concerns focus on development and behaviour, there is opportunity to collect information prior to the first visit.

- If reasons for the consultation only emerge when parents attend, it may be useful to collect information whilst they are in the waiting area.

The following information we have found useful in our clinical practice, collected either on paper (e.g. PDF questionnaire) or web-form. This has involved exploring a balance between too brief (information inadequate, not very helpful) and too lengthy (they tire). Open-ended questions about parents' worries are important, noting whichever concern is most prominent. It is also valuable to ask what they and others like about their child including strengths and interests.

1. **Information from parents about the family**

   - Demographics (for your records systems).

   - Arrangements and composition. If parents are separated this is an opportunity for you to share your policies on working with separated families.

   - Family history (medical, developmental, mental health).

   - Whether there is discussion they would prefer to have without the child present.

2. **Information from parents about the child**

   - Description of the child's interests, abilities, what the family likes about the child.

   - Summary of concerns.

   - What they would like to understand better about their child from the consultation.

   - What they would like help in managing.

   - A brief medical and developmental history

3. **Information from school.** If it is known beforehand that the consultation is for development/behaviour concerns, it may be possible for parents to ask the school (e.g. class teacher) to complete a brief questionnaire. Provided this is succinct and requested respectfully, compliance is generally high. Teachers have a vested interest in understanding and helping the children in their classroom, especially those with behaviour problems.

   - Description of the child's interests and abilities.

   - Summary of concerns.

- ○ What help the school would like (from the doctor).

- ○ Current supports provided by the school.

- ○ Copies of reports of standardized assessments.

4. **Information from other providers** (past and present). It is best for parents to ask for relevant information from other providers. This provides consent and also supports the parents' responsibility to contribute to the assessment.

Useful information from other providers includes:

A description of the child's problems and needs as they understand them to be.

A description of past and current services they are providing, including what they are working to achieve.

All previous assessments, letters, reports.

Standardized information

When it is known that child behaviour is a central concern it is best for parents to complete a standardized and validated behaviour questionnaire in addition to the individualized information above. Some examples of these questionnaires are described in Appendix 3.1. It is best to start with a broad-range behavioural questionnaire rather than one which presupposes a particular diagnosis.

Having the parents complete such a questionnaire before you meet with them has a number of benefits

- ◆ It saves a good deal of time in ascertaining the symptoms of behaviours and/or emotions of concern.

- ◆ Because questionnaires cover a broad range of symptoms, behaviours may be identified that might not otherwise arise in conversation. Parents may not appreciate these to be important or relevant. For example, the parents' spontaneous report may focus on their concerns about disruptive behaviours such as aggression. However, the child may also have symptoms related to anxiety or struggles with learning which may be important in management.

- ◆ Behaviours are described in language which has been tested for test-retest and interrater reliability. In other words, different reporters are likely to understand the description of the behaviour similarly.

- The questionnaire provides a valid record of the child's behaviour at the time of completion. This then forms part of the child's medical history. It is often helpful years later, for example when consulting about an adolescent's behaviour, to be able to look back and see whether symptoms are long-standing or not. This is far more reliable than parents' memories.

- Norms are available for some measures and may be stratified for different levels of developmental/intellectual disability. This means the severity of the child's behaviour problems can be compared with the general population of children with intellectual or other developmental disability.

- Key behaviours can be identified which can serve to monitor outcomes. The questionnaire serves as a baseline measure. This will be described further in the treatment Chapters 5 and 6.

In addition to general behavioural questionnaires, additional tools may be appropriate when particular problem areas are suspected from the referral (Appendix 3.2). For example, a number of questionnaires for the evaluation of Attention Deficit Hyperactivity Disorder (ADHD) are available

It is best to begin with a broad-range questionnaire as this does not presuppose any diagnosis. Questionnaires directed to specific diagnoses can always be added as guided by the clinical situation.

Inviting the family

It is common in standard paediatric consultations that only one parent attends. When the issue is child development and behaviour, however, both clinical assessment and ongoing management are much more likely to be successful if all parenting adults are involved as early as possible. Participation of relevant members of the extended family (e.g. siblings, grandparents) is valuable as early as possible in the clinical journey.

If you know that their concerns are about behaviour before you meet them, it is best to invite all family members to the initial consultation. If you discover the problem is a complex developmental/behavioural matter during the initial meeting, then the invitation can be made to invite other family members to a subsequent consultation. It is useful to develop a written policy that informs the family that it is in their child's interest that the paediatrician meets both parents, as that aids in understanding the child's problems. The emphasis is that it is in the child's interest rather than the doctor's preference. It is our experience that most parents respect the thoughtfulness and integrity behind this request, appreciating the doctor's desires to do the work well.

When children are moving between households following parental separation, some parents may not wish to be in the one room at the same time. You may need to make arrangements for them to attend at different times. From the outset, you need clarity regarding how they work together, particularly how they manage medical information (consultation letters, appointment requests) and how important decisions are made.

Chapter 1 discussed the 'time challenge' of doing this work well. Complex developmental/behavioural problems require different time and practice methodologies compared with standard paediatric medical practice. This is necessary for good practice rather than optional, just as the necessary time, instruments, and pre- and post-operative care are necessary for a specialized surgical procedure. Experience shows that setting up clinical care properly from the start not only leads to more successful outcomes but also greater clinical efficiencies in the future. Time spent initially is likely to be time saved later.

Managing the consultation

As you begin a consultation, there are several considerations that may help to set up the conversation. These clearly depend on the child's age and developmental level, and current mood state, such as their level of anxiety.

It is useful initially to discuss with the child and family how you intend to proceed. In a standard medical consultation this is usually straightforward. When the issue is behaviour, however, they may be uncertain what to expect.

Every doctor will have their own style to greet, introduce, and begin the consultation conversation. It is advantageous to have the child present from the outset and address the child early. By addressing the child first, you are showing the child from the start that you regard them as important. As appropriate to their developmental level, they can be reassured from the beginning that everything of relevance will be discussed with them. Any decision taken, as appropriate, will be with their consent. They will not be a passive observer of discussion by adults about them, especially not criticism of them.

The sequence of conversations: Who and when

The following is a suggestion only. The main need is to let those present know how you intend to proceed.

- Start with everybody together for initial exploration of the issues. In many consultations concerning children with developmental disabilities, the whole of the interview can proceed with everybody together.

- Sometimes it's necessary to talk to parents alone (e.g. if there are matters, they do not wish to discuss in front of their child).

- It may be desirable to talk to the child alone (e.g. for teenagers who have issues they do not wish to talk about in front of their parents).

How you address the material (what you are likely to achieve at what visit)

- When relevant, you may wish to share specific issues with them; for example, you can explain that it may not be possible to complete the assessment and make recommendations in one consultation, depending on the complexity of the material. At the end of the consultation, you will let them know how the process is should proceed.

Guidelines to negotiate early

As conversations regarding child behaviour may be 'uncharted territory' for the family and child, it is best to determine a set of 'ground rules' that guide how you will work together. For example:

- The purpose of the conversation is to understand and help (the child). To do this you need to ask questions that may be challenging, but the reason is to help you to understand the issues.

- In your consulting room, the child will not get into trouble. Even if you discuss problem behaviours, the purpose is to understand, not to blame or punish the child. The child needs to know that they are safe from blame and consequences within the consultation process.

- Privacy and confidentiality (e.g. what information you will keep private, what will be documented, and what you are required to disclose to parents).

- People see things in different ways. To understand the situation in the best possible way, you will be talking to everybody and hearing what they have to say. Everybody's view is heard and valued/respected. However, they may not agree with each other.

Opening conversation about the clinical concern

From the child's perspective, a conversation about their behaviour is often threatening. For further information on this a useful text is Encounters with Children by Radesky and Kistin (1). The following are some ideas to help them with these concerns.

Finding out the child's expectations

What does the child expect? What have they been told? You can find out by asking the child directly. The following needs to be modified to be understandable taking into account the child's developmental disabilities.

The child: *'I am going to talk to Mum and Dad in a minute, but can I ask you first—What did Mum and Dad tell you is the reason for coming to see me?'*

The child may be uncomfortable with this question. The child may have been told nothing or that it is just a doctor's visit.

If they struggle to answer the question, the parents can be asked:

> *'May I ask what you have told (child) is the reason you have come here today?' 'What is he expecting us to talk about?'*

Child: About the doctor

Children may have certain expectations regarding what a doctor does and talks about, then become upset when you talk about their behaviour. It may help to broaden their expectations:

> *'I'm a children's doctor. As well as helping children who are sick, I also help children who are finding things difficult, children and families who have upsets or worries.'*

Child: Reassurance about the process

Depending on the age of the child, they may have common fears that can be pre-empted.

Young children: *'Even though I am a doctor, I won't be giving any needles or doing anything that might hurt you.'*

Older children: *'If we talk about anything that you find too difficult or you feel embarrassed about in front of your parents, please tell me.'*

Child: Specific reassurance

As the conversation approaches issues of child behaviour, the child needs to know that they are safe.

> *'I have a rule in this office. If we talk about your behaviour, it is so we can understand. My job as a doctor is to find out what is hard for you and to help you. You are not going to get into trouble here.'*

Starting positively

You may consider beginning the conversation on a positive note. You may have written information about the child's strengths and interests that you can refer to:

'I like to start by getting to know children. What is fun for you? What do you enjoy? I've heard you're good at football. Your Mum has written here that you enjoy dancing. Is that true?'

And so on.

Talking about the presenting concerns

You may choose to begin with the child:

'Do you have any upsets or worries that you'd like me to help with?'. Of note, the term 'upsets or worries' is understood by children from a mental age of about 3 years.

'My job is to help children who find things hard. Can you tell me what you find hard?' (At school, home, as indicated by the child's age and presenting concerns.)

Beginning with the child has a number of advantages:

1. You reinforce to the child that you regard their view as important.

2. You find out initially what the child sees as the problem or problems before this is altered by hearing what their parents have to say.

3. You are seeking the child's consent to discuss their issues.

4. You can determine initially if they have any commitment to changing or improving things.

5. By showing the child that you think their views are important, you are telling the child that you are not just another adult who wants to hear how naughty they have been.

At this point the child may respond in a number of ways. The most straightforward way is that they may say 'yes', agreeing that you can talk to them, and you could ask them what their worries are, and the child may tell you. Commonly the child may just shrug their shoulders and look to their parents to provide some response.

If the parents jump in too quickly and want to say their views of what the child's worries are, you can politely tell the parents that you'd like to hear what the child has to say first. Then give the child enough time to decide.

If the child then is not able to suggest that they have any upsets or worries, then you can say *'well, is it OK if we ask Mum and Dad if they have any upsets or worries about you?'*

This question also has a number of purposes:

1. You would like to hear what the parents' concerns are.

2. It signifies that you are mindful of the child's consent to have the parents talk about them and their behaviour. Usually, the child will assent to your asking the parents to talk about their worries.

However, sometimes the child will say 'no'; that is 'it is not OK for you to ask my parents'. What does one do then? The child has not given consent for the interview to proceed.

This dilemma can be resolved by considering consent in the general paediatric setting. Up to the age of 14, generally speaking, the child's consent to medical intervention is not required if the parents consent. Therefore, when this problem occurs it can be resolved by putting the issue to the parents by saying, for example:

> *'It seems that (child's name) does not want us to discuss these concerns. How would you like us to proceed?'*

This enables you to see how the parents respond, exploring their parenting behaviour. The parent may say, for example:

> *'Well, I guess we can't proceed. We'll have to go home.'*

Such a response tells you a good deal about who has power in the house and the parents' lack of capacity to set boundaries and limits. A healthy parenting response would be to say something like:

> *'Well, (child) I understand you're not happy about us talking about it but, we're here to try to get some help for our family, so we need to talk about it. We'll continue to seek the doctor's help by discussing it.'*

The family's priorities

It is valuable to note exactly what the child and the parents state initially as their primary concerns. This is what is foremost in their mind. You may wish to write down their exact wording because it's useful to come back to this first statement at the end of the interview to ensure that you have addressed their presenting concern in the way they have perceived it.

In summary, the phase of 'setting up' your clinical conversation is important. It sets the stage, the purpose, the terms of reference, and a respectful style that optimises successful clinical work. The next step is to find out more about the child's behaviour.

The language disordered/non-verbal child

When children are unable to speak or unable to express themselves appropriately, consider their experience, what they hear and observe. They may understand more than is apparent from the outset. If in doubt, assume the child can understand rather than not.

Behavioural history

History to this point—the child's story

As in medical history taking, consider how current problems began and developed over time. For behavioural problems, what is this child's story?

◆ When did this begin?

◆ How did it get to this point? Has it been episodic, continuous, fluctuating?

◆ What has been done in the past to manage things and what happened?

In our experience, asking the child's story not only provides useful clinical information but it also serves to build the therapeutic alliance and trust. It is likely that the story may communicate a journey that has been very difficult for parents, perhaps one where they may also have experienced considerable guilt and shame.

Medical history

The medical perspective is both unique (within the network of professionals involved) and important.

◆ When considering past history and physical examination, you are looking for possible aetiologies for current dysfunction, before, during, or after birth.

◆ When considering the child's current state of health (review of systems), you are looking for medical factors that may influence the child's function in general, and behaviour in particular.

In addition to possible causal factors, medical history includes information regarding the problem and how it has been managed. In addition to medication, this includes behaviour management plans and their implementation, and psychological and therapy interventions.

When medication has been used, taking a history is similar to taking a behaviour history. You need to know what happened, rather than the child's or parents' *interpretation* of what occurred. To say that a medication did not work, or caused problem side effects is not the same as finding out the dosage, duration, consistency of usage, and direct information of subsequent behaviours. It may be that there was a problem with usage which, managed differently, still opens the option of using that medication successfully.

Current behaviour

To understand child behaviour, it is necessary to obtain the most precise description about the behaviours as possible. This enables you to know exactly what the child is doing and begin to understand why they are doing it.

A common mistake is to accept at face value an 'interpreted' history, which includes interpretative descriptors such as angry, impulsive, aggressive, intentional, and so on. Instead, a behavioural history enables you to know what happens as if you were watching (and listening to) a video of the behaviours directly.

There are various ways you can obtain a behavioural history. Following are approaches which assist the paediatrician to get an accurate history of the behaviours. Where there are a number of problematic behaviours, these questions are needed for each of the problem behaviours.

Information from completed questionnaires

If the family has completed a structured behavioural questionnaire, you may wish to start with behaviours recorded as most significant, then ask for more information about them.

For example, if the complaint is of aggression, one needs to know exactly what the aggressive behaviour comprises.

- **Action:** What do they actually do? Is it throwing objects, hitting people, spitting, punching, or kicking?

- **Observed emotions (affect):** Was the child unaware of themselves or their surroundings, (as in a seizure)? Were they excited, angry, sullen? Did they appear to be relating to outside stimuli (as in a hallucination, or in a dissociative state)?

- **Course:** What precedes and potentially triggers the behaviour? How long does it last? For how long does the aggressive behaviour continue? How rapidly does it develop? How does it terminate? Does it end suddenly, as it might with a complex partial seizure? Or does it gradually diminish until exhaustion as in the rages seen in Prader–Willi syndrome and hypothalamic injury?

♦ **Complexity:** Was the behaviour sufficiently complex that it could only be achieved with planning? Was it 'spur of the moment', reactive, impulsive?

Parents or carers will often reply with their theories about what is causing the behaviour or with generalizations about the behaviour. To get the conversation back on track, you can politely redirect the parents:

> *'I would like to come back to your thoughts about what is causing the behaviour, but at this point I am asking for a description of the behaviour itself.'*

To do this, it may help to change the perspective. For example:

> *'If I were a fly on the wall when this was happening what would I see?' 'If I were watching a video that recorded this, what would I see and hear?'*

ABC analysis—the sequence of events

A-B-C refers to Antecedents-Behaviour-Consequences. This is a basic but important component of assessing behaviour. It is mostly applied to fairly discrete episodes of behaviour disturbance.

Antecedents: This is a description of the circumstances immediately preceding a behavioural outburst, meltdown or 'escalation'. This allows you to identify possible 'triggers' of the behaviour, especially if there is a repeated pattern of antecedent. For example, a child with autism and hyperacusis has a meltdown whenever they enter a noisy environment, or when they are prevented from accessing their preferred activity.

Behaviour: This is the precise, sequential description of the behaviour as noted above. One needs to know not only exactly what the child does but how long it lasts. Further, what terminates the behaviour?

Consequences: Consequences are the responses to the behavioural episode of both the child and those managing the child.

○ The child: They may respond to their behaviour with apparent remorse if it has been an impulsive act which they regret. Or they may respond with apparent satisfaction if they have created a 'scene' which they find exciting, such as the arrival of the police.

○ Those managing the child: If the child has a tantrum when they are not given what they want, and the parent seeks to end the tantrum by providing what the child wants, this will have the effect of rewarding and reinforcing the behaviour.

Contextual variation

There is nearly always some variation in circumstances or context in which the behaviour is more likely or less likely to occur. Our term for this is **contextual variation**. Understanding this variation builds a more comprehensive picture of factors that contribute to the behaviour. It is also helpful in suggesting causal hypotheses which can be tested.

Sometimes it is obvious: for example a child with autism who has an intense drive to indulge some repetitive behaviour becoming distressed when they are prevented from carrying it out. Often, however, factors which are driving the behaviour are not clear. It is common to hear that the behaviour occurs unpredictably, seemingly at random.

Contextual variation helps illuminate this. You can explore the question by asking those who spend time with the child:

'When do you think the behaviour is more likely or less likely to happen?'

Commonly there will be different views about this from each reporter. This might reflect actual variations in behaviour in the different circumstances in which the reporter observes the child, or it may reflect different perceptions of the same behaviour. Look for any concurrence of opinion across the various reporters.

There are many contextual factors which can influence the likelihood, frequency, or severity of the behaviour problem. Some common ones are that the behaviour is more likely:

- With some people than with others

- At certain times of the day, week, or month

- In certain places

- In particular environmental circumstances, for example noisy places or busy places, or the opposite—very low stimulus situations

- At school or after-school care

- At home

- At the respite care facility

- When the drive to carry out a ritual or 'obsession' is frustrated

- When not given what the child wants

- When some other limit is imposed

Whatever time it takes to collect this information about contextual variation is worthwhile because this is the most useful way of generating hypotheses to explain the factors which are contributing to the behaviours. Such information can be valuable towards more effective and circumstance-specific interventions.

> ## Practice tip: Behaviour which is said to be unpredictable
>
> The degree to which behaviour problems are unpredictable is inversely proportional to the time spent looking for predictors!

Some reporters insist that behaviours are entirely random and unpredictable. This makes it very difficult to generate hypotheses about what is causing behaviour. You may need to emphasize to the family that you can't treat the problem with a successful response without first understanding what factors are contributing to it, and you need the family's help to do this.

Behaviour record (simple diary)

One strategy is the use of a behaviour record/diary. In our experience, this is most likely to be successful if the family understands the purpose and they have a strategy they consider achievable. The format and nature of information to be collected may need to be individually tailored.

We suggest a minimum of three behavioural episodes is necessary for information to be useful. A simple format is a single page of paper for each behavioural episode with headings and spaces to write responses. For each episode, minimum information should include:

- Date, time, and location.

- The circumstances in which it happened. Where were they? Who was present? What was happening immediately before?

- Exactly what happened.

Teachers can contribute to the diary, particularly if the child is in a specialized educational environment. They are likely to be motivated towards building understanding that leads to a more successful teaching experience. Recording information in a standardized manner may also help them learn to observe and understand behaviour with greater objectivity.

In addition to gaining more accurate information about contextual variation, completing a behavioural record demonstrates to the family that they have a role to play in understanding the behaviour. They learn to be more objective and analytical before jumping to conclusions.

Functional assessment

Functional assessment is a popular model applied to behaviour. It begins with a hypothesis regarding why the child might be doing what they do. Behaviour problems are regarded as being motivated by any of four 'functions'. These are to avoid difficult or unpleasant tasks or to escape stressful situations, to gain access to activities or objects they find safe and enjoyable, to gain attention, or to satisfy a sensory 'need'.

Understanding the function of behaviour from the child's perspective can provide clues to management approaches. These functions have been characterized in different ways by psychologists and there are a number of questionnaires specifically designed to elucidate these functions.

- The Motivation Assessment Scale is widely used despite evidence of limits to its reliability and validity.

- The Questions About Behaviour Function rating scale[1] has been shown to have adequate psychometric properties.

- The Functional Assessment Screening Tool (FAST) provides questions for a semi-structured interview.[2]

Assessment of each behaviour

The behavioural assessment methods described above need to be undertaken for each behaviour problem separately, or as appropriate for groups of similar behaviours, self-injurious behaviour, damage to property, etc. The factors contributing to one behaviour problem may be very different from those contributing to a different behaviour problem in the same child.

Direct assessment of the child

Each paediatrician develops their own style of child assessment. Some may be formal, others non-directed and play based. Strategies vary according to circumstances, particularly child age. A key component of paediatric assessment

---

[1] https://arbss.org/wp-content/uploads/2021/05/Questions-about-Behavioral-Function-QABF-Google-Docs.pdf. (2000). Accessed 3 March 2024.

[2] LaRue R. Functional Analysis Screening Tool. In: FR Volkmar (eds), *Encyclopedia of Autism Spectrum Disorders*. New York, NY: Springer; 2013. https://doi.org/10.1007/978-1-4419-1698-3_1141

is to develop an intuition or 'feel' of the child beyond any formal data gathered. Communicating emotion is more difficult if consultations are undertaken using telehealth/video methodologies. For assessment related to child behaviour, at least one early face-to-face appointment is recommended if possible. This is because the reports of others do not always align with direct impressions gained by interacting with the child.

The issue arises about whether to talk to the child by themselves or whether to talk with the child in the presence of the parents. It is generally best to start with the whole family and then the interview can be flexible after that. This decision is usually clearer after meeting the child and family. If talking to the child by themselves is likely to be too difficult for them, there is nothing wrong with continuing to interview the child with the family present.

Talking to children is a core skill for paediatric doctors. The methodologies described below are suggested only. In particular:

1. The child probably knows the conversation relates to their behaviour. They may be defensive. Some ground rules should be made explicit. Examples are that the child is safe, that it is your job to understand and help them.

2. Adjustment to the child's developmental limitations. As paediatricians gain experience, this becomes intuitive. If a child has an intellectual disability, you adjust to their presumed capacity (developmental age-equivalent). If they have receptive language problems, you shorten and simplify your language. If their social comprehension is impaired, you limit your assumptions regarding the degree to which they understand the perspective of others.

It is best to begin with a conversation that recognizes where the child feels positive about themselves. It makes a difference if they understand that you see what they are interested in, good at, care about, the positive aspects of their life. Where children are strongly engaged in online games or social media learning what they do serves to collect important data as well as form a connection with the child.

Some specific strategies may assist. One is the 'Three Wishes' question: 'If I were a magician and I could grant you whatever you want' ('whatever you would like to change' is sometimes a useful phrase), 'what would be your three wishes?' Those three wishes often reflect what is most important in the child's mind. If the child's wishes are solely for objects, it may suggest a level of emotional deprivation. At younger mental ages, material objects are perceived as a way of replacing emotional deprivation. The child may respond by talking about certain changes in their life circumstances or their family interactions, which of course is valuable in helping you to understand what matters to the child.

The conversation with the child is another opportunity to understand the child's perspective on any behavioural difficulties that have already been described by other family members. How do they understand themselves, what they do, and why this occurs?

Mental state

Assessment of mental state is a routine part of training in psychiatry and psychology, but not necessarily in paediatric medical training. It involves a standardized set of considerations. In principle, it is equivalent to conducting a cardiac or neurological examination in physical medicine. It provides a standard structure for communicating what you observe intuitively.

During your time with the child, the following observations contribute to a mental state assessment:

- **Appearance and behaviour:** For example, do they look undernourished? Are they dishevelled? Do they appear passive, restless, distracted?

- **Speech and language:** What is the child's manner of speech, for example, noting echolalia, neologisms, or aprosody? Are they fluent with language? What is the sophistication of their vocabulary and grammar?

- **Mood:** What observations can be made about their affect? Do they appear frightened? Confident? Cheerful? Unhappy? And how do these mood states respond to your interactions? Are they able to be cheered up? What happens to their thinking if they become upset or angry?

- **Thought:** Does the child's conversation follow a logical stream? What disturbances in the child's cognition do you observe? How do they make judgements of cause and effect?

- **Socialization:** How do they interact? Do they engage readily with the assessor? Do they readily appreciate the possible perspectives of other people?

Family assessment

The set-up section above noted the importance of hearing all points of view regarding what may be going on with the child's behaviour. This section extends this discussion to consider evaluation of the family itself.

Assessment of children's behaviour requires assessment of the child's psychosocial world. Whilst this varies with each child, it generally includes direct family, others at home, school, and other community environments such as respite care and activity programmes.

In the consideration of family, it is best to include siblings from the outset. For children with disabilities, siblings may one day need to take care of their disabled brother/sister. The seeds of responsible future care are sown when all the children are young. It is reasonable, however, to interview both parents initially and then see the siblings at a later time.

There are many reasons for doing this. For child behaviour problems, involving the whole family from the outset is more likely to enable a successful understanding and management pathway. You will be able to determine

- **Parental mental health**: Are there any mental disturbances/disorders in parents that may be inherited by the child, or impacting how parents manage the child?

- **Each parent's story**: What have they experienced, especially when they were children? How might this impact their parenting?

- **Multiple perspectives**: With behaviour problems there is usually no single perspective on cause or course. Everyone has their opinion. The siblings also have their own view on the disabled child's behaviour problems. '(Child) has meltdowns when Mum and Dad fight'.

- **Family roles**: What is each family member doing to support/hinder the child with the developmental disability?

- **Family beliefs**: What are the different perspectives within the family, for example who is blaming whom? Who is feeling ashamed or guilty? What is the impact of the behaviour problem on each family member? Do the siblings suffer survivor guilt? Does the family deny, minimize, or exaggerate the disability?

- **Culture**: What does the child's disability mean to a family of their cultural background?

Practice tip: The family is all those who have an important role in the child's life

One parent may assert that the other is not involved in the child's care. It is advised that this issue be explored rather than taken at face value. To interview one parent and not the other is like examining the chest and not examining the abdomen! Likewise, if grandparents or others have a strong role in a child's life, invite them to attend also.

Genogram

A genogram is a very useful tool in family assessment and is recommended as a routine procedure. Genograms serve multiple purposes:

- They provide a visual image of the people in the child's family and their relationships.

- They encourage the paediatrician and the family to consider the roles of extended family members.

- They potentially indicate intergenerational patterns of behavioural disorder.

- Genograms create a starting point for exploration of strengths and challenges in relationships between family members.

- They potentially identify people who can assist with management.

- They may improve understanding of cultural traditions in family relationships.

Interviewing the family

Interviewing in regular paediatric care works to understand the medical needs of the child. Interviewing families extends this to build an understanding of how the family system works in their care of the child.

Practical arrangements

Different systems of care may constrain how family assessment is undertaken. In Australia, for example, billing systems require the child to be 'in attendance'. That often means the child waits in the waiting room whilst doctors talk to parents.

This can be challenging for children, who may wonder what is being said about them. As noted above, regardless of the arrangements, it is best to inform the child exactly what is going on, what you will be talking about, why you are doing this, and what you will let the child know about what is going on when they are not present.

As appropriate and needed, you may need arrangements that to talk to:

- Parents alone and together

- Child alone

- Siblings either alone or with parents

- Grandparents, if they are actively involved

The paediatrician's perspective on the problem: Multidirectional partiality

When there are a set of discrepant views expressed by different family members about the behaviour, the paediatrician has to be neutral, at least in the assessment phase. If not, the unaligned parent will see you as an ally of the other parent and will write off/disregard your opinion promptly. This risk may be obvious particularly when parents are separated and uncooperative but is also important when parents hold different views about the child's problems.

Beyond maintaining neutrality, a more active role for the doctor is 'multidirectional partiality'. This means that you show each family member that you understand (are partial to) their view. Whilst you show that you understand, that does not mean that you necessarily agree. The easy way to show multidirectional partiality is by repeating back what each person says, usually rephrased. The intended outcome of this is that both parents feel understood, and that they regard you as a perceptive paediatrician. For example:

DOCTOR: *'So, what do you think gets him angry?'*

MOTHER: *'Freddy gets angry when his father ignores him'.*

DOCTOR: *'So, I understand you feel child's behaviour is sensitive to Dad's attention?'*

MOTHER: *'Yes, that's right.'*

DOCTOR: *'And what do you think provokes the anger, Dad?'*

FATHER: *'Freddy gets upset when Mum doesn't give him what he wants, because she spoils him.'*

DOCTOR: *'I see. You feel that a problem is not setting limits on Freddy's demands?'*

FATHER: *'Yes, you've got it.'*

This intended strategy of multidirectional partiality can extend to your discussion with the siblings, adjusting the language to suit the children's ages. For example, the child with the disability is 10 years old. His younger sister Mary is aged 4, and older brother James, aged 12, have both come along to the interview.

DOCTOR: *'Mary, what do you think makes Freddy upset?'*

MARY: *'When James yells at him.'*

JAMES: *'No, mostly he gets stressed when Mum and Dad are arguing.'*

This process of actively listening to each perspective can extend to the next level, in which you find out what each family member's views are about the others' opinion.

DOCTOR: *'So, what do you think Dad, about Mum's view that he's sensitive to your attention?'*

FATHER: *'Well maybe, but that's a minor factor.'*

DOCTOR: *'And what do you think Mum, about Dad's view that the anger is about not getting what he wants from you?'*

MOTHER: *'Yes, it's hard to say no, but he dotes on Dad.'*

DOCTOR: *'It sounds like you agree that both factors play a part.'*

MOTHER AND/OR FATHER: *'Yes, I think you're right, Doc.'*

Non-attendance by a family member

As noted above, where possible, it is best to invite all parents from the outset. Even with these efforts, however, it is common that one parent, usually the mother, attends with the child and not the father, even when there is a father involved in the child's care.

When enquiring about this, a common response is that the father is too busy and is unavailable. However, fathers are generally able to be available if they choose to be, if they consider it of sufficient importance. There are many options you can offer them. They can join by video or phone or attend at a time that suits them.

The child's mother may indicate that the father is not interested or doesn't like talking to doctors. When involved parents or family members choose not to attend there are several strategies to consider.

- **Via the mother**: Suggest to the child's mother that it is not possible for you to fully understand the child without hearing the father's point of view. The father's perspective is critical before you are able to progress.

- **A direct request (e.g. email)**: for example 'Dear Mr Jones, I've been seeing your son in regard to the school's concerns about his behaviour there. This is an important problem, and I would very much appreciate hearing your thoughts about how we can help him. Please contact my office to make a time that suits you so I can hear your suggestions....'

In our experience, a personal request such as this usually increases the likelihood of getting the child's father along. It is very difficult for a father to accept that their opinion about their child's needs is unimportant.

When the father does then come, much will be learned about family function. Sometimes, the father is very interested in the child's behaviour and the mother may have kept him away from the consultation, fearing it would threaten the paediatrician's support for the mother's viewpoint. Less commonly, it may be that the mother's account of the father seems accurate. That is, they take little interest in his child's problem. There are numerous other variations on these possibilities.

Information from other sources

The more sources of information, the greater the likelihood of understanding the nature of the child's behaviour. It also provides an understanding of the beliefs and strategies currently adopted by those, such as teachers, who manage the child.

Selecting which sources, and what to find out from each source, may be a clinical judgement based on individual circumstances.

School

It is common that parents bring the child for paediatric consultation because of complaints about behaviour at school. In this case, discuss with the family that it is not possible to provide input about school behaviours without talking to school staff directly.

If your practice knows that the child's behaviour is an issue at school, it would be helpful to collect simple written information from the child's teacher before the initial consultation. A simple strategy is online forms or brief PDF questionnaires that parents can print and ask the teacher to complete.

After meeting the family, it is likely that you would wish to obtain further information from the school. How such information is obtained will depend on local circumstances and relationships.

It is better to talk directly with the child's teacher and other staff involved. Where possible, arrange a school case conference (see Practice tip in Chapter 5). Alternatively, a video or telephone call may suffice. In situations where arranging this proves to be difficult, it is helpful to talk with the school Principal. If they appreciate your interest and the importance of sharing information, they generally can make these conversations happen.

With written information there are a variety of strategies you can explore:

- **Narrative information**: Sometimes teachers find it easier to share their experience of the child's behaviour, and to express their views about what needs to be done, in response to open-ended questions rather than a standardized assessment.

- **Standardized behaviour assessments**: Reports about behaviour from school are much more useful if they include structured reports, for example the Developmental Behaviour Checklist-Teacher Version or Connors Teacher Rating Scale.

♦ **Standardized developmental assessments**: The school may be able to share cognitive, language, or other relevant assessments, particularly if the child has educational services dependent on evidence of developmental diagnoses.

Information you may wish to gain from the school includes:

♦ **Education context**: Which type of school or schools has the child attended? Has the child been in a regular class or a special education setting and of which type? What supports are provided? What professionals, either within or outside the school, do they work with?

♦ **Strengths**: What do they see as the child's more endearing qualities, their strengths and interests within the school setting?

♦ **Concerns**: What do they worry about? What do they find difficult to manage? What would they like assistance with?

♦ **Hypothesis**: Do they have an opinion regarding why the child is behaving as they do?

♦ **Strategy**: How are they managing behaviour at the moment? What seems to be working?

♦ **Anything else**: You may not have asked about something they consider relevant. Is there anything else they would like to share, that may or may not be important?

The relationship between parents and school is important. Is it constructive or dysfunctional? What is the school's attitude to children with disabilities? Some schools are very rigid in their expectations and have little tolerance of a child who is different. Others are quite flexible.

Bullying

Bullying at school is an issue that requires special attention. Unfortunately, it is very common and has serious adverse consequences for the child. The child may be the recipient of bullying but may also be a perpetrator. Child, parent, and school perspectives on this are important, as they are frequently at odds. Assertions about 'who started it' are usually not helpful. What matters is what the school is doing about it. There needs to be a strategy for the bully and for the victim as well as a whole-of-school approach.

Out-of-home care and respite care

Children in out-of-home care, or attending respite care, often have significant developmental problems, and these are commonly associated with behaviour problems.

For adolescents, information may also come from activity centres, supported employment, or work experience. Here again, it is useful to obtain reports of behaviour from validated checklists in addition to unstructured comments from carers, both in writing and direct conversation.

The key point is that the more settings that can inform you about the child's behaviour, the better you will understand the child's behaviour.

When seeking information from these facilities, it is best to request it from a person who knows the child well, and even better if that person has some authority, such as a house manager or team leader. Your time invested in negotiating with the person in authority will be well repaid when it comes to asking the manager to ensure ongoing cooperation with your management strategies.

Chapter summary

This chapter examines clinical assessment in time sequence:

- Referral, and what information may be reliably gathered prior to initial consultation

- Initial consultation, setting expectations, and defining processes

- Defining the behaviour

- Assessment of the child (medical, developmental, behavioural, mental health)

- Assessment of the family (history, face-to-face)

- Other sources of information (school, out-of-home, and respite care)

- Putting assessment information together into a diagnostic formulation

Where appropriate, specific information is provided regarding assessment methodologies specific to understanding child behaviour. An example is the assessment of family, the importance of multiple perspectives, and dealing with non-attendance of key family members.

Appendix 3.1

Questionnaires to assess a broad range of behaviours

There are a number of questionnaires aiming to cover a broad range of behavioural and emotional disturbances and designed for use in the neurotypical population which can be used with children with milder developmental disabilities. For further information on questionnaires, we recommend.

Assessing and Diagnosing Young Children with Neurodevelopmental Disorders A DSM-5-TR Compliant Guide, 2025, by Nicholl (2).

All the questionnaires described below have well-established psychometric properties. These can be explored further through the links provided.

General population questionnaires

These questionnaires are designed to cover a broad range of behavioural and emotional disturbances. They have been devised for use in the neurotypical population, which can include children with milder developmental disabilities. These questionnaires can be used both as a brief and convenient overall measure of disturbance severity as well as monitoring treatment progress.

Strengths and Difficulties Questionnaire (SDQ)

The SDQ is designed as a behavioural screening questionnaire for children and adolescents aged 2 to 17 years old. It has 25 items describing symptoms. These can be supplemented by questions measuring the impact of the symptoms on distress and function. A further follow-up form assesses change in symptoms over time.

There are self-report (completed by the youth), parent-report, and teacher-report versions. Population norms are available from Europe, Australia, and the United States.

- Cost: free

- Languages: 80

- Clinical use: brief broad range behaviour survey

- Further information: sdqinfo.org

Child Behaviour Checklist (CBCL)

The CBCL is a 106-item questionnaire which forms part of the Achenbach System of Empirical Behaviour Measurement (ASEBA). Versions are available for preschoolers and school-age children. Forms for the school-age group are a parent-report form, teacher form, and a self-report form for adolescents.

The CBCL provides a detailed account of emotional and behavioural problems as individual behaviours, syndrome subscales, and overall severity and DSM diagnosis screens. The CBCL can be used to monitor progress as well as inform assessment. The questionnaires are scored as a Total Behaviour Problem Score, two broad-band scales (internalizing and externalizing behaviours), and as eight syndrome subscales (Aggressive Behaviour, Anxious/Depressed, Attention Problems, Rule-Breaking Behaviour, Somatic Complaints, Social Problems, Thought Problems, Withdrawn/Depressed). The CBCL also produces DSM-oriented scales which screen for DSM diagnoses.

- Norms are available from many countries

- Languages: 90

- Further information and cost: aseba.org

Questionnaires specific for children with developmental disabilities

Developmental Behaviour Checklist (DBC)

The DBC (3) was designed to assess a broad range of emotional and behavioural disturbance in children with developmental disabilities. It is modelled on the CBCL but the items are different. The team who put this together includes Professor Einfeld, author of this book. It can be used for detailed description and measurement of behaviour problems as well as monitoring of treatment outcomes. Use for monitoring outcomes is discussed in Chapter 5 (Appendix 5.1).

There are versions for children aged under 4, 4 to 18, and adults, and for completion by teachers. There is also a short form, the DBC-S. The DBC can be scored for the Total Behaviour Problem Score, or five subscales: disruptive, self-absorbed, communication disturbance, anxiety, and social relating. There are separate norms for children with mild, moderate, and severe/profound intellectual disability. There is a monitoring version to measure treatment outcomes.

- Norms: Australia, Finland, United Kingdom, United States

- Languages: 21

- Further information and cost: Wpspublish.com/dbc2

Aberrant Behaviour Checklist (ABC)

The ABC (4–6) is intended to assess a broad range of problem behaviours of children (and adults) with developmental disabilities. It has 58 items which are grouped into five subscales: Irritability, Social Withdrawal, Stereotypic Behaviour, Hyperactivity/Noncompliance, Inappropriate Speech

- Norms: United States

- Languages: 35

- Further information and cost: https://www.slossonnews.com/ABC.html

Appendix 3.2—Tools for specific diagnosed conditions

We expect paediatricians to have an understanding of tools appropriate for their clinical setting and practice. Specialized assessments are available to assist with the evaluation of specific disorders, including those below:

- **Autism:** Autism Diagnostic Observation Scale, Autism Diagnostic Interview, and Childhood Autism Rating Scale.

- **Anxiety, Depression, and Mood:** ADAMS (7), Spence Anxiety Scale. The SCARED (Screen for Child Anxiety and Related Emotional Disorders). The ADAMS measures manic and depressive mood, anxiety symptoms, and compulsive behaviour in subjects over 10 years old with all levels of intellectual disability.

- **Attention Deficit Hyperactivity Disorder:** Vanderbilt, Conners.

- **Cognition:** Mullens Scales, Griffiths, Bailey Scales, IQ tests, Kaufman Brief Intelligence Test.

- **Language:** Clinical Evaluation of Language Fundamentals, Peabody Picture Vocabulary Test, Preschool Language Scales.

- **Learning:** WIAT, WRAT.

Specialized assessments are also available for specific developmental functions, including

- **Executive functions:** Behaviour Rating Inventory of Executive Function.

- **Specific academic skills:** Reading assessments (e.g. Neale), CTOPP (Comprehensive Test of Phonological Processing).

- **Social competencies:** Social Communication Questionnaire, Social Skills Rating System.

Appendix 3.3—Cases

Case 1. Jack

As with medical 'differential diagnosis', there is a set of information you would like to find out from Jack, his family, and school. This was discussed in Chapter 2.

Discussion

How would you assess possible contributors to Jack's behaviour?

From Jack directly: Much information can be obtained through informal conversation. The paediatrician will be able to observe his level of social engagement and maturity, his self-control, his language comprehension and expression, and capacity for insight into his situation. What does he think is the problem? What does he want, and what does he believe can be changed?

The use of standardized questionnaires can be very helpful, such as the Achenbach, Strengths and Difficulties Questionnaire, and ADHD questionnaires. Standard information from multiple sources (parents, teachers) not only provides information about Jack but also about the observer, and where information agrees and differs.

From the family: Much of the information is likely to come from Jack's family. In addition to their answers to questions, the paediatrician will be able to observe how they interact with Jack. Presuming the foster father is involved, it is of major importance that they attends at least one of these sessions. The foster father's perspective is important, and you will be able to observe how he and his partner interact. It is generally important to clarify the nature of the fostering arrangements, what resources are available, what decisions can be taken by the family without reference to relevant authorities, and so on.

From the school: For multifactorial problems that include significant school contribution, parent report as well as written information from school is often not enough. Jack's situation is not only problematic but likely to be worsening over time. Direct methods of communication with schools may include a phone call, video teleconference, or even face to face case conference.

* If you are able, it is best to book a time to talk with the most relevant professional at the school (teacher, principal, special needs coordinator). It is helpful to send them (e.g. email) a list of issues/questions you would like to discuss beforehand, so they are best prepared.

- Case conferences, either video or face to face, are the most effective method for communication and collaboration. These work best with a clear agenda and chairing structure (see Practice tip in Chapter 3).

- Sometimes you need to contact schools during the consultation. When calling schools, it is best to be firm and not easily deflected. If it is not possible to talk with the teacher at that time, ensure there is an arrangement that enables this important conversation to occur reasonably soon.

Case 2. Jade

Jade is a 14-year-old girl in her second year of high school. She has a diagnosis of high-functioning ASD made four years earlier. Her behaviour has been worsening over the last 12 months, with angry, non-compliant behaviour at home and school avoidance.

You consider it likely that there are multiple contributing causes in addition to her ASD. These may include her lifestyle (sleep, gaming, social media), her struggle at school (peer relations, organization and completion of work), and factors in family life (e.g. her father is described as 'similar, rigid', often losing his temper with Jade's behaviour).

Discussion

Based on your hypotheses of possible cause, how might you go about assessing her, her family, and school?

The paediatrician's relationship with Jade is critical, based on trust and respect from the outset. To achieve this, it is necessary to be patient and listen, to understand the world from her point of view and validate this as appropriate. She is suffering underneath the blanket of problem behaviour.

It is possible Jade has a form of Executive Dysfunction that results in disorganization, and reduced capacity to manage the multiple curricula demands of school. This is examined through history (current and past) as well as standardized questionnaires. Where this is unclear, a neuropsychological assessment may assist.

If the information suggests a Specific Learning Disability (e.g. with maths), this may benefit from psychoeducational assessment.

It is likely that Jade's social limitations impact relationships with peers. Does she have friends? Is she being bullied, including social exclusion behaviours? Evaluation of this comes from discussion with the school, Jade's parents, and Jade herself.

In assessment of the family there are several important questions to examine. What are the perspectives of her mother and father? What are the family rules? How do these differ by parent, including how they are managed. How do they protect the younger boy? More generally, how is the family faring? How is the marriage, the mental health of each parent, financial health, and sense of support (e.g. extended family)?

If Jade has an Individual Learning Plan at school (or equivalent), it is likely that there is an individual teacher who coordinates this. A phone call with that person may be a good place to start. How do they make sense of her struggle, her behaviour, and how do they manage these (particularly the school avoidance)? How well is her curriculum adapted? How do they manage bullying?

For Jade, are there unique considerations regarding how to go about assessment?

It is important to keep Jade informed during every step of the way, particularly when talking with the school. If Jade finds out the paediatrician has been discussing her 'behind her back', there is significant risk that trust will be lost.

It is also important to include the whole family (particularly her brother) in the process. There are possible family interactions that the paediatrician needs to understand. An example is Jade's potential perception that her brother is favoured in the family. This may have a basis in reality or may not. This will be readily apparent with brother's participation in the interview, but obscure without it.

Case 3. Alfred

Alfred returns to see you at age 9 years. He has Down syndrome and moderate Intellectual Disability (ID), and his mother and teachers are concerned he has ADHD. He is hyperactive, impulsive, and has a very short attention span. He is in a self-contained class of ten children with two teachers. He is demanding of attention but there are no major concerns regarding his moods or aggressive behaviour. The family history of ADHD and substance abuse is noted in his father and older brother. Vanderbilt rating scales from both parents and teachers meet symptom criteria for ADHD.

Discussion

What additional information might be helpful to you in this assessment?

It is clear that Alfred has symptoms of ADHD across settings, but is the severity of inattention and hyperactivity/impulsivity beyond what is expected for a child with moderate ID, who is functioning at the 4 to 5 year age level? It may be helpful to get the teachers' perspective on this. Also, to what extent are these symptoms causing additional functional impairment for Alfred? To what extent are they causing parenting stress? You may also want to engage Alfred in informal play or structured tasks, providing an opportunity for observing task persistence, motor activity, and executive functions.

References

(1) Radesky J, Kistin C, eds. *Dixon and Stein's Encounters with Children. Pediatric Behavior and Development*. 5th ed. Elsevier; 2025.

(2) Nicholl N. *Assessing and Diagnosing Young Children with Neurodevelopmental Disorders A DSM-5-TR Compliant Guide*. 2nd ed; 2025. https://www.routledge.com/Assessing-and-Diagnosing-Young-Children-with-Neurodevelopmental-Disorders-A-DSM-5-TR-Compliant-Guide/Nicoll/p/book/9781032933108

(3) Einfeld SL, Tonge BJ. The Developmental Behavior Checklist: The development and validation of an instrument to assess behavioral and emotional disturbance in children and adolescents with mental retardation. *J Autism Dev Disord*. 1995;25(2):81–104.

(4) Aman MG, Singh NN, Stewart AW, Field CJ. The aberrant behavior checklist: A behavior rating scale for the assessment of treatment effects. *Am J Ment Defic*. 1985;89(5):485–491.

(5) Stoddard J, Zik J, Mazefsky CA, DeChant B, Gabriels R. The Internal Structure of the Aberrant Behavior Checklist Irritability Subscale: Implications for studies of irritability in treatment-seeking youth with autism spectrum disorders. *Behav Ther*. 2020;51(2):310–319.

(6) Kaat AJ, Lecavalier L, Aman MG. Validity of the aberrant behavior checklist in children with autism spectrum disorder. *J Autism Dev Disord*. 2014;44(5):1103–1116.

(7) Esbensen AJ, Rojahn J, Aman MG, Ruedrich S. Reliability and validity of an assessment instrument for anxiety, depression, and mood among individuals with mental retardation. *J Autism Dev Disord*. 2003 Dec;33(6):617–629.

4

Diagnosis or diagnostic formulation?

What's your hypothesis?

Following a comprehensive bio-psycho-social assessment (Chapter 3), the paediatrician has a set of information regarding the behaviour, the child currently, their current world, and their past experiences. What is the best way to assemble and organize this information to provide an efficient explanation for the behaviour?

In medical practice, it is traditional to make a diagnosis. For children with developmental disorders and problem behaviour, however, the explanatory utility of diagnosis is incomplete. This is due both to limitations in describing developmental disability as well as describing behaviour.

Our proposed resolution of these limitations when assessing a child to understand their behaviour is the use of diagnostic formulation rather than diagnosis.

Further reading: Types of diagnoses used in developmental paediatrics

Aetiological diagnoses—diagnoses based on causation

- **Causal:** The diagnosis describes a biological mechanism of causation, for example Fragile X syndrome.

- **Inferred:** The diagnosis describes a causal process for which there is strong likelihood based on known biological mechanisms and the individual's history. However, causation remains inferred rather than certain, for example Fetal Alcohol Spectrum Disorder.

- **Past experience based:** The diagnosis requires past child experience in addition to, as well as presumably causing current symptoms, for example Reactive Attachment Disorder, Post-Traumatic Stress Disorder (PTSD).

Clinical diagnoses—diagnoses that characterise clinical problems but make no causal assumption

◆ **Quantitative:** The diagnosis requires statistically as well as clinically significant deviation in degree from the norm, measured with validated tools, for example Intellectual Disability (ID), Developmental Language Disorder, Specific Learning Disability (SLD), Attention Deficit Hyperactivity Disorder (ADHD).

◆ **Qualitative:** The diagnosis reflects symptoms which are qualitatively abnormal, irrespective of degree. For example, psychotic disorders are categorically abnormal.

How clinically defined diagnoses are constructed

Categorical diagnoses reflect a 'top-down' approach to categorization. By consensus, a diagnosis is agreed to exist. Diagnostic criteria are then determined. The outcome is that a child either has the diagnosis or doesn't. The criteria used to diagnose Autism Spectrum Disorder (ASD) are an example.

Dimensional diagnoses are derived through a bottom-up methodology. Symptoms are measured in the population. Statistical methods are used to identify co-occurring symptoms and to identify which level of symptoms is clinically important. One example is the system developed by Achenbach, derived from the statistical evaluation of empirical data (e.g. the factor structure of questionnaires such as the Achenbach Child Behaviour Checklist).

In practice, most are mixed: The symptoms of some disorders are abnormal by degree, but when the severity crosses a threshold, they are considered categorically abnormal. Autism and Anorexia Nervosa may be considered as examples.

Systems of diagnosis

The Diagnostic and Statistical Manual, 5th Edition (DSM-5) (1) and International Classification of Diseases, 11th Edition (ICD-11) (2) are accepted by consensus as official diagnostic classifications. ICD-11 intends to cover all disorders, whereas DSM-5 only classifies mental disorders. The DSM system is developed by the American Psychiatric Association, whereas the ICD system is developed by the World Health Organization.

It is important to understand that before any criteria for a specific mental disorder are considered, the general requirements for diagnosis of any mental disorder need to be present. Although there are different definitions of mental disorder in the literature, the DSM requirements are commonly used. These requirements are:

- **Abnormal symptoms or signs:** These can be qualitatively abnormal, for example hallucinations; or quantitatively abnormal, such as motor overactivity.

- **Distress:** The symptoms cause distress to the individual or to others in the community.

- **Impairment:** The symptoms must result in significant compromise to the child's function.

For example, a child may be anxious and distressed about attending school, but that is not sufficient to make a DSM diagnosis of an anxiety disorder. However, if the anxiety results in significant school non-attendance, they may have an anxiety disorder.

There are also a number of exclusions in applying a diagnosis of mental disorder. For example, the diagnosis of mental disorder cannot be based on sexual or political preference. The reader is encouraged to read the introduction chapters of the DSM-5 manual for further information on these issues.

Mental disorders in the presence of intellectual disability

There are two specialized diagnostic systems to address mental disorder classification in people with ID.

1. The Diagnostic Classification—Learning Disorders (DC-LD) (3), developed in the United Kingdom (where the term Learning Disorders refers to Intellectual Disability). This is an adaptation based on ICD diagnoses.

2. The Diagnostic Manual—Intellectual Disability (DM-ID) (4) developed in the United States. This is an adaptation of the DSM classification.

Both of these classification systems propose diagnostic criteria for mental disorders which take into account the reduced communication and conceptual abstraction capacities of children and adults with ID.

Limitations of diagnosis in developmental paediatrics

The purpose of diagnosis is to describe the condition and communicate that information in an understandable and meaningful way. The problem in practice is that many of the diagnoses used in developmental paediatrics may not do this very well.

Table 4.1 compares the medical diagnosis of appendicitis with two common diagnoses used in Developmental Paediatrics, Oppositional Defiant Disorder (ODD) and ASD.

Information inherent to diagnoses

Below are some of the reasons why the information provided by individual diagnosis may be limited. This may not be a comprehensive list.

- **Complexity of the causal mechanisms.** The brain is an incomparably more complex organ than the appendix vermiformis. All the factors contributing to the emergence of behaviour problems described in Chapter 2 are complex individually and collectively. Describing these phenomena with a single or several diagnostic labels is likely to be simplistic.

- **Uncertainty about causal pathways.** It was once thought that scrofula and pulmonary consumption were two different diseases. When the tubercle bacillus was shown to cause both, the diagnosis of tuberculosis became a much better descriptor. We do not have good knowledge about many causative mechanisms.

- **Within-category** heterogeneity: Two children with the same diagnosis (e.g. ASD) may have very different clinical challenges due to individual differences for both severity and pattern of component problems. See comment in Table 4.1. This heterogeneity is particularly true for child behaviour

- **To lump or to split?** That is the question. A child has a disorder and some of the symptoms are a part of that disorder and also seen in another disorder. Some doctors will diagnose two separate disorders, and some will combine into a single inclusive diagnosis. This issue frequently presents in ASD as 'obsessions' and potentially other anxiety-driven phenomena are a necessary criterion for the diagnosis. Should the clinician diagnose ASD alone, or should they diagnose Obsessive-Compulsive Disorder (or another form of anxiety disorder) in addition to the ASD? Another example is the restrictive eating pattern often seen in autism. Does the diagnosis of ASD cover this, or should they also be diagnosed with Avoidant/Restrictive Food Intake Disorder (ARFID)?

In clinical practice, the answer to the lump or split problem is often what is best for the child. If additional diagnosis allows the child to be understood better, or to access beneficial therapy, then multiple diagnoses are clinically justifiable. This is why a clear profile of impairment is necessary for each child.

Table 4.1 Limits to information provided by diagnosis

	Appendicitis	ODD	ASD
Signs and Symptoms	Nearly always the same.	Vary by reporter, intensity and comorbidity.	Highly variable across most domains. 'When you've seen one child with autism, you've seen one child with autism' (5).
Agreement on diagnosis between doctors	High.	Relatively poor agreement between doctors, because doctors rank the significance of overlapping conditions differently, for example conduct disorder, disruptive mood dysregulation disorder, anxiety disorders, intermittent explosive disorder.	Reasonable agreement at the ends of the severity spectrum, but greater disagreement about 'borderline' cases.
Course and prognosis	Very clear.	Unpredictable. Some get worse, some get better, some stay the same.	Lifelong disability, but severity of impairment fluctuates across different domains, with intervention efficacy and degree of environment adaptation.
Underlying pathology	Consistent and clear.	Contribution to cause comes from a large potential array of variable factors, often unclear.	Hundreds of different genetic and other causes but mostly idiopathic.
Sociocultural factors	Little difference across societies and countries.	Major cultural differences in behavioural norms.	Unclear because of differences in diagnostic practices.

(Continued)

Table 4.1   Continued

	Appendicitis	**ODD**	**ASD**
Treatment	Appendectomy is nearly universal.	Variable need for and efficacy of different classes of psychotropic drugs, different types of psychological therapies for the child and the family at home and at school.	Variable indications for different classes of psychotropic drugs, different skill-building therapies with significant disagreement about intensity, duration, etc. Varying need for allied health interventions.
Conclusion	The diagnosis 'Appendicitis' says almost everything one needs to know about the condition.	The diagnosis of ODD puts the current symptoms in the ballpark of behaviour that upsets and disrupts. That's about all it tells us.	The diagnosis of ASD says the child will have an uncertain degree of lifelong impairments in social communication and restrictive behaviours. That's about all.

◆ **Binary responses to dimensional psychopathology:** When a cut-off is imposed on a dimension, a patient who scores just below the cut-off and a patient who scores just above the cut-off will be classified differently, but in practice they are clinically indistinguishable. Further, the patient who scores just above the cut-off may be classified the same as a patient whose score vastly exceeds the cut-off, although they are clinically very different.

An example in developmental paediatrics is the DSM-5 diagnosis of ADHD. The criteria state: 'Hyperactivity and impulsivity: symptoms have persisted for at least six months to a degree that is inconsistent with developmental level.' Some children will be only slightly deviant from developmental level, while some will be extremely deviant. How deviant is enough to make the diagnosis valid?

This problem is not restricted to developmental paediatrics. A child with a Body Mass Index (BMI) of 29.9 is classified as overweight, whereas a child with a BMI of 30 will be classified as obese. However, there is no significant difference in the health risks for these two children. On the other hand, a child with a BMI of 45 will have far greater threats to their health than the child with a BMI of 30, but they will both receive the same classification as obese.

> # Practice tip: Is a diagnostic label enough?
>
> You may have a good understanding of a child, but how much information does your diagnostic language, on its own, convey? Consider a letter you have written from the perspective of the reader. If you have not discussed the child further, to what extent does the diagnosis documented in the letter communicate what is necessary to understand and manage the child?

Additional risks inherent to diagnosis

A number of risks potentially arise when clinicians are required to respond to diagnostic uncertainty and complexity with diagnosis.

Diagnostic overshadowing

Diagnostic overshadowing refers to the tendency of clinicians to incorrectly ascribe behaviour problems of people with diagnosed disorders to the disorder alone. Using the example of ID, this thinking ascribes the behaviour to ID, rather than considering the behaviour disturbance as comorbid or contextual. The bias that results potentially leads to under-assessment and under-treatment (6).

Major behavioural disturbance occurs in about 40% of children and adolescents with intellectual disability (7). Whilst this figure is high, it also means that the majority (60%) of children and adolescents with intellectual disability do not have major behavioural disturbance. This suggests that intellectual disability itself does not cause problematic behaviour. For the 40% there is some factor other than the ID itself which is causing or substantially contributing to the behaviour problem.

An exception is when the behaviour is typical for the child's developmental age. A physically large 15-year-old adolescent with severe ID may have a developmental age of 2 to 3 years. If that adolescent has temper tantrums, these could be considered typical for children of the same developmental age. The behaviour is problematic, however, due to the 15-year-old's size as well as expectations that the child think and behave at chronological rather than developmental age

Confirmation bias

Confirmation bias refers to the tendency to search for, interpret, favour, and recall information in a way that confirms or supports one's prior beliefs or values (8). A common example when children have ID is the belief that children have purpose behind their behaviour that is not actually present.

Impairment

In addition to imprecision of diagnoses, there is imprecision regarding how impairment attributable to the diagnosis is evaluated. At the time of writing there were no studies of the interrater agreement of ASD levels of support listed in DSM-5. In Australia, clinicians are required to state these levels for children in funding applications. This is the likely explanation for the increase in diagnosed prevalence of ASD Level 2, with a corresponding decrease in Level 1.

Medical diagnoses attribute all to the child

By definition, a diagnosis characterizes information presumed in most cases to be inherent to the child. This is true even when the origins may have been external, such as Reactive Attachment Disorder. When associated with child behaviour, diagnosis may imply the full explanation of the child's behaviour rests with the child. Using diagnostic terminology to explain child behaviour overlooks the interactive, environmental, and contextual factors that also have a strong causal influence on the child's behaviour.

Advantages and disadvantages of diagnoses

Advantages

- Validates to parents and others that problems are 'real' and do not arise from child intention and choice alone.

- Communicates to parents, teachers and clinicians the broad nature of the child's problem.

- Often required to access financial and therapeutic supports, for example insurance coverage for some services may be contingent upon documentation of a diagnosis.

- Provides information regarding the type of adjustments needed. An example is the modification of communication for a child with a Developmental Language Disorder.

- Guides access to further information and support organizations.

Disadvantages

- May provide little information to explain the sources of the behaviour.

- May provide little to inform management.

- May result in inappropriate treatments. This is a risk particularly for 'spectrum' diagnoses with a wide range of clinical expression. Treatment may be directed to the diagnosis rather than the individual needs of the child. This may occur both with professional services as well as 'Dr Google' treatments.

- May stigmatize the child in the minds of others.

- May impair the child's self-esteem or self-concept (they believe there is something wrong with themselves).

- May imply lifelong impairments when such cannot be accurately predicted.

Both advantage and disadvantage

- 'Medicalizes' the problem, relieving the parents of responsibility. It does, however, provide access for the doctor to become involved in management of the behaviour.

Diagnostic formulation

We will use the terms 'Diagnostic Formulation' and 'Formulation' as synonymous. Applied to child behaviour, formulation is the process of combining all the key information about the child into a structured summary explanation of their behaviour.

Practice tip: Understanding why

'Do not ask which disease the patient has. Rather, ask which patient the disease has!' (William Osler). This expands thinking beyond the diagnosis to consider the patient as a whole. Diagnostic formulation works towards that goal, by addressing the question 'Why is the child behaving in this way?'

There are a number of ways of structuring a formulation. Each of these is an attempt to organize and structure a broad set of factors that contribute causal understanding. In this case, the formulation is specific to understanding a child's behaviour problems.

Different formulation structures may be appropriate for different clinical purposes. An example is the multi-axial structure of mental health diagnosis in DSM-IV, removed in the transition to DSM-5 (9). Bespoke formulation strategies have been proposed for developmental paediatrics (10) generally. It is probable that experienced clinicians have developed their own approach to the collation and communication of clinical complexity.

The effort, and benefits, of learning and using formulation

To begin with, formulation may represent an additional layer of workload for the busy clinician. With time, however, it becomes a source of efficiency. As information is acquired through the assessment process, formulation provides a meaningful place to locate and organize the information in real time, as it is acquired. Once assessment information is complete, the formulation framework provides a succinct overview of diagnostic information that is able to directly guide strategies of management.

Table 4.2 Properties of diagnosis compared to formulation

	Diagnosis	Formulation
Construction	A succinct word or phrase to describe a disease.	A structured collation of all information arising from assessment, which contributes to understanding the child's behaviour.
Length	Concise.	Expanded as needed.
Standardization	The diagnostic term ideally has measured properties of validity and reliability.	The structure can be standardized, however the contents are unique to the child and clinical circumstances.
Derivation	Based on consensus, or broad acceptance across the profession.	Determined by the individual medical practitioner for the individual patient.
Scope	Diagnosis generally describes issues intrinsic to the child.	Formulation extends beyond the child to include relevant factors of the child's environment.
Range	Diagnosis is limited to capturing the content of the diagnostic criteria.	Formulation is an overarching structure for including an unrestricted range of relevant information, for example, across time and location.

Formulation for child behaviour: The 5P model

For the assessment and management of behaviour in children who have developmental disorders, we recommend a '5P' approach used in mental health (11), adapted for child behaviour. We have found the "5P" structure to be useful, reliable and relatively simple.

The 5Ps are influences named **predisposing, protective, precipitating, perpetuating,** and **palliating.** Predisposing and protective refer to background risk (behaviour is more or less likely to occur). Precipitating, perpetuating, and palliating refer to the time sequence of the behaviour itself.

Predisposing

Predisposing refers to identifiable factors that **increase the risk** of problem behaviour.

- **Child:** Even if a cause (such as brain damage or genetic lesion) has not been demonstrated, developmental disorders are likely to have an organic aetiology. The resulting impairments could be considered predisposing factors. How do brain problems reduce the child's capacity to behave as expected and increase the likelihood of problem behaviour? They may have difficulty managing their emotional responses to perceived threat and uncertainty. They may have trouble comprehending, they may misunderstand, or struggle to use language to negotiate.

- **Environment:** What is happening currently in the child's world that increases the likelihood of problem behaviour? The child may be feeling unsafe due to bullying or problems at home.

Managing predisposing factors (e.g. pharmacological treatment of ADHD) alters the likelihood of the problematic behaviour occurring. An example is the child with impulsivity who, with the assistance of medication, has greater opportunity to think, remember and consider consequences before acting.

Protective

Protective factors **reduce the risk** of problem behaviour, especially in otherwise vulnerable children. The importance of identifying protective factors in a diagnostic formulation is that these are potentially factors that can be utilized and strengthened in a treatment programme.

- **Child:** What properties of the child reduce the likelihood of difficult behaviour? They may find certain activities interesting and motivating. They may enjoy interacting with people. They may have the capacity to solve problems in difficult situations effectively.

- **Environment:** A nurturing family is protective. A compassionate, understanding teacher and school are protective. There may be others who like the child and understand and adapt to their needs. There may be places where the child is happy and engaged. A known, predictable and stable environment is likely to be protective.

Precipitating

What situations initiate a process where this behaviour is likely to occur? Reducing immediate triggers is likely to reduce frequency and intensity of behaviour.

- **Child:** What are triggers for the child? These may be fatigue, confusion or misunderstanding, sudden noises, or perceived anger in others. Unexpected change in routine is a common trigger for autistic children, as is being denied a preferred activity.

- **Environment:** What circumstances overwhelm the child, triggering difficult behaviour? These may be changes the child is not expecting, or requests experienced by the child as aggressive. It may be sudden, unexpected noises (for example, hand dryers).

Perpetuating

After the child commences problematic behaviour, what identifiable factors increase the likelihood that that behaviour will continue?

- **Child:** What makes it hard for the child to change behaviour once the behaviour problem has begun? It may be hard for them to settle emotionally, to negotiate verbally, or to believe in the goodwill of those who they are otherwise able to trust when they are calm.

- **Environment:** What may be observed that makes it difficult for the child to settle? It could be overwhelming activity and noise. Behavioural instruction may be experienced by the child as unachievable, harsh, unsympathetic, or unreasonable. The child may see no face-saving resolution pathways. Is the behaviour rewarded, as the child perceives it? The way behaviour is managed may serve as 'secondary gain' for the child.

Palliating

What identifiable factors increase the likelihood that the behaviour problem will settle and resolve?

- **Child:** The child may settle down if they are easily redirected to an enjoyable activity, or in the presence of a trusted adult, such as loving parents or a valued school teacher. They may settle if their perspective is heard and validated.

◆ **Environment:** Properties of the environment that assist settling behaviour include clear and practised pathways to manage difficult situations safely, catching problems early, before they escalate, opportunities for the child to settle in safety, with dignity, and the presence of a trusted adult.

The value of a 5P approach

The 5Ps comprise a model to help us think broadly about possible factors contributing to a behaviour problem.

In putting the model together, a single factor may be relevant to **several** of the model's components. It is not necessary to critically allocate each contributing factor to just one of the Ps. For example, the child with a history of child abuse may have disturbed attachment and volatile, heightened threat response. These can be considered both predisposing and perpetuating.

Balancing diagnostic rigour with flexibility

Diagnostic systems and taxonomy of diagnoses is our best attempt to understand and classify our patients' conditions. DSM and ICD diagnoses of mental disorders are often approximations supported by current consensus. A diagnosis may not be set in stone but could often be considered a working hypothesis, subject to change as new evidence accrues.

It is important for the clinician to maintain appropriate rigour in applying diagnostic criteria. The degree to which this may be necessary varies according to health care systems. It may be, for example, a prerequisite for prescribing medications approved in the treatment of specific diagnoses.

At the same time, the clinician should understand the limitations of diagnosis and maintain some flexibility. It may be more clinically meaningful and therapeutic effective to describe and understand a child's behaviour than to rely just on a diagnostic label.

The limitations of formulation

Formulation is a way of organizing multifactorial information as it informs the issue to be understood. It is only as good as the information that goes into it. The validity and utility of formulation will reflect the quality of the assessment process and the experience of the assessor. If the assessment process has been superficial, then the resulting formulation will be correspondingly limited in clinical utility.

Formulation plus diagnosis?

It is often advantageous to provide both a formulation as well as a diagnosis to describe the behaviour problems. A well-considered formulation is always helpful but it may not be sufficient, particularly when access to understanding, supports and services is diagnosis-dependent.

Putting it all together

How are contributory factors mapped into an efficient diagnostic formulation? We recommend this mapping be undertaken in real time rather than after the assessment, and suggest an approach undertaken in three steps: (1) to summarize the behaviour effectively, (2) to consider the child, and finally (3) the environmental contributing factors.

Behaviour

From the assessment information identify several key components of the behaviour. These form a basis from which change due to intervention can be measured:

1. What the child does (says, actions) as observed rather than interpreted information:

   ○ Frequency and severity of these behaviours.

   ○ Why this behaviour is a problem for the child (Chapter 1).

   ○ Why this behaviour is appropriate for medical attention (Chapter 1).

2. Patterns and properties of the behaviour that map onto the precipitating/ perpetuating and palliating aspects of formulation:

   ○ How the prevalence and severity vary with changes in environmental context.

   ○ What starts the behaviour.

   ○ What appears to keep the behaviour going.

   ○ What is effective in settling the behaviour down.

The child

Predisposing

◆ Current problems of health and/or safety.

◆ Limitations in the child's capacity (current competencies, the impact of the child's developmental disorder) to manage expected normative behaviours or behaviour challenges, especially where there is brain pathology.

◆ Temperament/personality properties such as sensitivity and social competency.

◆ The child's past, how this may have been internalized and exerts continuing influence on the present. In these cases, the child's central nervous system responds to current challenges as if they were the same as past experience.

Protecting

◆ Strengths, talents, and other resilience factors, including temperamental factors.

Precipitating

◆ Demands the child is unable to understand or meet.

◆ Stressful environments, for example a noisy place for a child with hyperacusis.

Perpetuating

◆ Responses to the behaviour that the child cannot understand or manage.

Palliating

◆ Properties of the child that respond to certain strategies (e.g. desire to be heard, soothed, clarity of direction).

The child's world

In a similar manner, there are identifiable properties of the child's world that either increase or decrease the likelihood of problem behaviour, as follows.

Predisposing

◆ An unsafe or volatile environment (e.g. domestic violence, bullying).

◆ A neglecting environment with insufficient capacity to meet the child's needs (e.g. poverty, family stress).

◆ An environment that does not understand the child's individual competencies, or has not adapted appropriately to this understanding.

◆ An environment that either models or more directly encourages the difficult behaviour.

Protective

◆ Environments that are flexible, with the capacity to consider and meet the child's needs.

◆ Environments that care, putting the time and effort into necessary adaptations and supports.

◆ Networks of care (e.g. home and school) that collaborate effectively.

Then, for the behaviour events themselves:

Precipitating

◆ What is it about the child's world (physical, sensory, social) that triggers behaviour?

Perpetuating

◆ What in the child's world keeps the behaviour going? Is it a lack of place to settle with safety and dignity?

Palliating

◆ What in the child's world helps them calm down: who, where, how?

> ## Practice tip: Through the child's eyes
>
> With assessment information organized into an efficient formulation structure, you should be able to see the world as the child sees it, as through their eyes. Instead of the child's behaviour being an enigma, understanding enables an 'of course' response. If you were that child, in that situation, the behaviour makes sense. You may well do that behaviour yourself.

Chapter summary

Although diagnosis is a powerful tool in general medicine, it has limitations when applied to understanding developmental disorders generally, and problem behaviour specifically.

◆ Different diagnoses communicate variable levels of information, particularly due to within-diagnosis heterogeneity.

◆ Individual diagnoses may only explain part of the child's situation.

◆ There are multiple diagnostic types. Diagnosis may refer to a medical finding (e.g. genetic), clinical patterns related to past history (e.g. Fetal Alcohol Spectrum Disorder (FASD), PTSD), or patterns of current clinical findings without clear and identifiable causation.

Diagnostic formulation is a recommended structure that extends diagnostic categorization to address three additional dimensions:

1. Child-specific factors that have a direct influence on behaviour (increase or decrease likelihood).

2. The child's environment (biopsychosocial influences); and

3. The time sequence of behaviour itself.

The formulation structure proposed has five components (5P model):

1. Factors that alter the background likelihood of this behaviour occurring.
   - Those that increase the risk (predisposing)
   - Those that reduce the risk (protective)

2. Factors specific to behavioural episodes.
   - Those that trigger the behaviour (precipitating)
   - Those that maintain the behaviour once it has begun (perpetuating)
   - Those that settle the behaviour once it has begun (palliating)

Appendix 4.1—Clinical cases

Case 1. Jack

From your assessment of Jack, his family, and school, it is clear that his behaviour arises from multiple contributing processes. He has trouble managing perceived threats, likely to interpret uncertain social situations as threat. His family struggles to manage his behaviour effectively. Peers at school have a mixed response to what is likely to be socially immature behaviour. His school is unable to adapt fully to his individual needs in curriculum, social, and behavioural support. Jack has little insight into his own situation. He is developing the belief that he is not liked, but he feels unable to change.

You need an efficient way to put this information together in order to help others understand the causes of Jack's behaviour as well as to guide management planning.

Discussion

To what extent do you consider the diagnoses of FASD/ADHD sufficient to explain Jack's behaviour?

A diagnosis of FASD sends a set of clear messages, most notably that the problems arise from toxic brain damage, the resulting impairments are significant and multiple and are likely to be permanent to a significant degree. This is a good start to understanding Jack's predicament.

The diagnosis of ADHD may not be so well understood. Some do not believe it at all, preferring to blame the child with assumptions of intention. There may be a belief that it is solely a 'medical' problem and medical treatment is sufficient to manage it such that behavioural strategy (at home, at school) is not necessary.

For both FASD and ADHD, the risk is that *all* causal attribution is directed to the child. Child-based diagnoses do not carry information about how the behaviour and challenges more generally are managed. In Jack's case, how he is managed is a critical consideration as no 'treatment' of Jack in isolation is likely to be successful.

If these diagnoses are not sufficient, how would you organize explanatory information into a 5P formulation structure?

Predictive factors include Jack's weaknesses in the context of situations where he struggles to manage what is expected. They may include specific challenges (e.g. reading-heavy subjects, team sports), or times of day when he is fatigued. Poor goodness of fit elevates background likelihood of problem behaviour.

Protective factors provide a path to build Jack's resilience and confidence. Are there activities he enjoys, where he feels successful, cared for, and appreciated? Are there people with whom he feels happy and safe (a grandparent, the school manual arts teacher)? Can hard things just be avoided, with protective activities instead?

Clarifying **precipitating** triggers leads to consideration of prevention. Are there certain subjects or situations more likely to set him off? An example is being asked, without warning, to contribute in class. At home it may be homework after a long day.

Perpetuating and palliating factors inform how behaviour is managed once begun. Can teachers be trained to talk gently, to reassure, to provide a face-saving path for him to leave situations? At home, is it possible to improve behavioural strategy with greater calm, clarity, and consistency? Does the family understand how hard it is for Jack to learn, such that behavioural strategy is not a 'quick fix'?

Case 2. Jade

Jade is a 14-year-old girl in her second year of high school. She has a diagnosis of high-functioning ASD made four years earlier. Her behaviour has been worsening across the last 12 months, with angry non-compliant behaviour at home and increasing school avoidance.

From your assessment you have determined multiple probable contributing causes. When not angry, Jade appears sad and unmotivated. As suspected, her sleep and lifestyle are becoming more disrupted, she is struggling at school with work completion, and relationships with peers and several teachers, who consider her rude and disrespectful. It is clear that her use of the Internet and social media is a big part of her life and identity.

Her father is spending more time at work, with much of Jade's aggression directed at her mother and brother. Her parents have differing perspectives on what is going on and how it should be managed. They are increasingly struggling to set and sustain boundaries for Jade and her behaviour.

You need an efficient way to put this information together in order to help others fully understand Jade's behaviour as well as to guide an integrated, co-operative path to management.

Discussion

For Jade, to what extent does her diagnosis of ASD explain the behaviour problems?

The goal is to understand why Jade is unhappy, school avoidant and difficult at home. Her ASD diagnosis communicates that Jade has trouble understanding social situations, including the experience, beliefs, perspectives, and feelings of others. It provides some explanation for her social struggle, including lack of respect or perspective-taking in how she makes sense of the world.

The diagnosis also communicates risk of associated problems (e.g. ADHD/Anxiety/SLD) but does not provide further information about this. It does not explain why she is angry.

The primary limitation of the diagnosis is that it provides little information on which to base management. Jade is likely to be unenthusiastic to engage with social skills capacity building. Even if she did, what difference would it make? The diagnosis does not guide either how much or in what way to adapt to her needs.

If the developmental diagnoses are not sufficient, what would you include in a 5P diagnostic formulation that you consider essential to understanding his behaviour?

Predisposing: Factors that increase the risk of school avoidance and angry behavioural episodes include her lifestyle (sleep, fatigue); weak social cognition; tendency to escalate emotionally when stressed; tendency to interpret uncertain social situations as threat; her inability to meet the social, academic, and organizational demands of school; and the inconsistency of behaviour management strategy at home. Marital discord at home may elevate her background anxiety. Her behaviour remains more likely whilst she continues to be angry (e.g. she is likely to feel devalued as an 'outsider').

Protective: When she is calm, Jade is able to use her intelligence and language. Her family loves her and wishes to help her. There are some teachers at school who are 'on her side'. She is happy and proud of herself when succeeding at what she loves.

Precipitating: Jade escalates quickly when she feels accused, controlled, or unable to meet demands to her own expectations or the expectations of others. When confronted with a difficult challenge (e.g. attending school), she is likely to avoid it in some way. She escalates more rapidly when she can see no path out of the situation, feeling trapped and humiliated.

Perpetuating: Jade 'digs in' when challenged, when spoken to firmly (she hears this as anger, disapproval), and when she perceives that others' demands to modify her behaviour are unachievable or just unreasonable.

Palliating: Jade settles down with the family dog, in her room alone (she has several activities that help soothe her that she enjoys). She has a good friend at school whom she talks to. At school there are teachers and activities where she feels safe.

Case 3. Alfred

Alfred is a boy with Down syndrome and moderate ID whom you last saw at age 9 years (Chapter 3). At that time, he was diagnosed with ADHD and started on stimulant medication. He showed moderate improvement on parent- and teacher-completed ADHD rating scales, and was discharged to primary care follow-up, doing well on extended-release methylphenidate 10 mg daily.

He is referred back to you at age 12 years because of concerns about his moods and behaviour. He is currently taking extended-release methylphenidate 30 mg each morning. Alfred is moody and irritable especially in the afternoons. He readily resorts to assaultive behaviour when he doesn't get his way, evident at school, at home, and at his respite facility. In addition, Alfred spends a good deal of time acting as a character from a particular TV soap opera. He often demands that his carers take on other characters from the show, and he sometimes becomes aggressive when they do not comply.

Alfred lives with his mother and usually visits his father on weekends, although these visits have become sporadic. He continues to be impulsive and hyperactive when he is with his father (his father does not give him the medication). He absconds when upset, demonstrating little understanding of danger.

His mother reports that Alfred occasionally witnessed domestic violence in earlier years reportedly perpetrated by his alcoholic father, but she has no concerns about ongoing abuse, direct or observed. General health has been good, other than recurrent otitis media and severe dental caries with prior periapical abscess requiring surgery.

You need an efficient way to put this information together in order to help others fully understand Alfred's behaviour as well as to guide management planning.

Discussion

What are Alfred's likely diagnoses?

Alfred's established diagnoses are Down syndrome, ID, ADHD, with possible Disruptive Mood Dysregulation Disorder and Dissociative Identity Disorder.

What are the potential risks to Alfred of only considering his diagnoses?

If the paediatrician were *only* to consider Alfred's diagnoses, management options may include increasing his stimulant (or 'topping up' the dose in the afternoons), and augmenting the stimulant with a mood stabilizer or antipsychotic medication. In our experience, stimulants may be helpful in low doses to treat ADHD symptoms in children with developmental disabilities, but benefits when doses are increased may be outweighed by side effects, including irritability. In this case, Alfred may already be experiencing the side effect of rebound irritability in the afternoons on the higher dose of methylphenidate, and his moods may improve when the methylphenidate is discontinued, or the dose decreased.

What would a diagnostic formulation based on the 5P model look like, and what does such a formulation add to your understanding of his behaviour?

Predictive factors include Alfred's cognitive and language impairment, and his high degree of impulsivity. Also, we have learned about previous traumatic events in which he witnessed domestic violence. He is biologically predisposed to misunderstand or misinterpret, to escalate emotionally in the presence of perceived threat and behaviour with 'flight / fight' purpose.

Protective factors provide opportunities to build Alfred's coping skills. His favourite activities are opportunities for recreation and positive engagement with others. He enjoys loving and nurturing relationships with both parents.

Precipitating triggers are most often not getting his way. This maladaptive pattern of behaviour has been reinforced over many years. Also, Alfred may be experiencing afternoon and evening rebound effects from his morning dose of methylphenidate. When he is uncertain, socially confused, or events unfold in an unpredictable way, his threat response escalates quickly with behavioural consequences.

Perpetuating and palliating factors focus on how Alfred's behaviour is managed. Can the behaviour strategies employed by his parents and his teachers be fine-tuned and more consistent?

A diagnostic formulation that considers the 5Ps, Alfred's capacities, and the important role of trauma provides the doctor with a broader understanding of Alfred. Sharing this understanding with his family, teachers, and carers is therapeutic, helping them to work effectively as a team, and informing a broader set of management strategies that go beyond prescribing medication. The two goals of sharing formulation information are (1) they understand Alfred to the degree that moves beyond comprehension to empathy and (2) the formulation provides a logical foundation for shared intervention strategy and goals.

References

(1) American Psychiatric Association. *Diagnostic and Statistical Manual of Mental Disorders: DSM-5*. 5th ed. American Psychiatric Association; 2013.

(2) International Classification of Diseases (ICD). World Health Organization. *International statistical classification of diseases and related health problems*. 11th ed. https://icd.who.int/; 2019.

(3) Royal College of Psychiatrists. DC-LD: *Diagnostic Criteria for Learning Disability: Diagnostic Criteria for Psychiatric Disorders for Use with Adults with Learning Disabilities/ Mental Retardation*. 1st ed. Royal College of Psychiatry Publications; 2001.

(4) Kastner TA, Walsh KK. Diagnostic Manual–Intellectual Disability: A Textbook of Diagnosis of Mental Disorders in Persons with Intellectual Disability, by R. Fletcher, E. Loschen, C. Stavrakaki, and M. First. *Intellect Dev Disabil*. 2009;47(4):323–328.

(5) Flannery KA, Wisner-Carlson R. Autism and education. *Child Adolesc Psychiatr Clin N Am*. 2020;29(2):319–343.

(6) Peña Salazar C, Arrufat F, Santos J, Fontanet A, González-Castro G, Más S, et al. Underdiagnosis of psychiatric disorders in people with intellectual disabilities: Differences between psychiatric disorders and challenging behaviour. *J Intellect Disabil*. 2018;24:174462951879825.

(7) Einfeld SL, Tonge BJ. Population prevalence of psychopathology in children and adolescents with intellectual disability: II. Epidemiological findings. *J Intellect Disabil Res JIDR*. 1996;40 (Pt 2):99–109.

(8) Nickerson RS. Confirmation bias: A ubiquitous phenomenon in many guises. *Rev Gen Psychol*. 1998;2(2):175–220.

(9) Substance Abuse and Mental Health Services Administration. DSM-5 Changes: Implications for Child Serious Emotional Disturbance [Internet]. Rockville (MD): Substance Abuse and Mental Health Services Administration (US); 2016 Jun. Available from: https://www.ncbi.nlm.nih.gov/books/NBK519708/

(10) O'Keeffe M, Macaulay C. Diagnosis in developmental–behavioural paediatrics: The art of diagnostic formulation. *J Paediatr Child Health*. 2012;48(2):E15–26.

(11) Macneil CA, Hasty MK, Conus P, Berk M. Is diagnosis enough to guide interventions in mental health? Using case formulation in clinical practice. *BMC Med*. 2012;10:111.

5

Management

It is a mistake to go direct from behaviour to prescription, bypassing assessment, formulation, and planning. It isn't just about pills!

Planning care

Planning management of behaviour problems in children with disability is guided by the same set of principles, regardless of the child's disability or the behaviour itself.

1. Address the safety of the child and others.

2. Address important issues of general health.

3. Base the plan on objective measures of behaviour and a diagnostic formulation that explains the behaviour.

4. Set priorities (child and family priorities, what is easiest to do, most likely to work early).

5. Consider intervention both around managing the child and the child's world (particularly family and school).

6. Decide who will do what (what can you do, referring and working in collaboration with others).

7. Set and evaluate outcomes.

8. Overview and case management.

Safety

Safety of the child

Is the child at risk of harm from the behaviour itself? Examples include absconding, running across a road, or undoing a safety harness while a passenger. Management may need to begin with physical boundaries such as car seat technology, gates, fences and locks.

Is the child at risk of harm from those around them? Is there a possibility of active, ongoing abuse (physical, sexual, emotional, neglect)? In such a case, the appropriate step is to ensure safety through child protection channels.

At a level below threshold for child protection intervention, the child's behaviour may still communicate a level of safety risk that demands intervention. This could be at home (e.g. domestic violence), school (e.g. bullying), or the child's mental health more generally (demoralization, despair, self-harm ideation). It is unlikely behaviour will substantially or sustainably change in the presence of ongoing threat or safety risk. When a child is not safe, behaviour may be their voice, such that it is harmful to silence that voice.

> ## Practice tip: Safety first
>
> No behaviour management strategy will be effective while the child feels threatened.

Safety of others

Danger to others includes harm (e.g. hitting) as well as **threat** of harm (e.g. holding up a knife). In more extreme cases it may be necessary to consider the child's behaviour as a form of assault such that management involves police for both prevention and response to behavioural incidents.

Successful management of the child's behaviour is unlikely whilst those around feel unsafe.

- If unsafe behaviour occurs at school, it is best to negotiate with school staff first regarding what is necessary for their safety and the safety of peers. For example, this may involve keeping the child away from school, or indoors at lunchtime.

◆ If unsafe behaviour occurs at home, the paediatrician should address this with the family as a priority (see Practice tip and Further reading). The family has a right to safety just as do the members of the school. It is not in the interests of the child or the family if aggressive behaviour is tolerated for reasons such as the child's disability and distress. Tolerance risks the child growing up using threats and violence to resolve their distress and get their own way.

Practice tip: Safety at home

If aggressive behaviours by others occur at home, for example domestic violence, it is unlikely an individual child will learn to control their behaviour in a healthy way. Precedents and examples from others provide a strong message about acceptable ways to solve problems.

Further reading: The safe family

When unsafe behaviour occurs at home, shift the focus from the individual child's behaviour (e.g. to stop aggression) to the family as a unit. This enables focus on a positive vision (the safe family). It enables discussion at a whole-of-family level. This can be addressed, for example, through a whole family discussion.

1. Do they want to live in a safe family? Why? What are the benefits for individuals when they feel safe? What are the benefits for the family unit?

2. What are the behaviours that cause family members to feel unsafe (the more specific the better)? This is not directed at any individual; they are applicable to all family members. These should be identified as specific observable behaviours (e.g. hitting another family member) rather than more general principles (e.g. not hurting). They define a 'safety boundary' for the family.

3. If individuals within the family behave in a way that falls outside the safety boundary, what happens? How this is managed will vary across families, but the guiding principles are that the consequences need to be immediate rather than delayed, and the message to the individual who crosses the safety boundary, communicated by the action taken, is that they effectively, temporarily lose the right to access full participation in, or benefits of family life. This is because the family is a safe place for all. The message is that they need to learn to manage their aggression in order to

enjoy the full experience of family. An example strategy is the child (1) in time out for a fixed period of time and (2) needs to identify and suggest a change to ensure a safe family before returning. Optimally they discuss what they could do instead in the same trigger situation.

4. How will the 'safe family' project be reviewed? When is the next family meeting? What will be discussed at that meeting?

Such planning requires the capacity of all members to understand and participate. There are many circumstances where this capacity is not present (e.g. the teenager with severe intellectual disability (ID)), and other strategies will be necessary to keep the family safe.

Safety of the paediatrician

It is not wise to risk injury from children who have the capacity to harm. Self-protective strategy may include having the child escorted, or consulting in a physical environment that enables preservation of professional safety.

Health

Assessment of the child's health is centrally important, particularly if the child is unable to communicate effectively and there has been an unexplained change in behaviour and/or function. If there is pain (e.g. ear, tooth, abdominal, joint) this needs to be addressed prior to any other behaviour management strategy. If the child is unwell, their capacity to modify behaviour is compromised by fatigue. This is discussed in further detail in Chapter 2 (Causes).

Diagnostic formulation

Management planning builds on the diagnostic formulation. In the previous chapter, the 5P approach to formulation was recommended.

Practice tip: Measure twice, intervene once

The more comprehensive the formulation, the greater the range of potential management strategies available to the paediatrician, and the more likely these are to be successful.

This informs management planning in two fundamental ways.

1. **Reducing background risk.** An understanding of the Predisposing and Protective factors informs strategy to reduce predisposing and increase protective contributing factors. Predisposing-informed strategies may include use of medication, working with the child through Cognitive Behaviour Therapy (CBT) and mindfulness, altering curriculum, bullying, and other sources of stress, building family cohesion and collaboration. Building protective factors may include better health and sleep, more time doing what the child enjoys, and more time with those who love and care for the child. Building the child's capacity to understand themselves and acquire new adaptive skills will reduce behaviour problems.

2. **Preventing and managing behaviour episodes.** Consideration of Precipitating factors leads to strategy intended to reduce frequency and intensity of predictable behavioural events. Triggers may include any of the contextual factors listed in Chapter 2, but examples are loud instructions, bullying from other children, the child not getting their own way, or misunderstanding social situations. Understanding Perpetuating factors informs strategy to minimize problems once behaviour has begun. A common example is to avoid talking in a confrontational way to the child, criticizing them, and trying to address the triggering situation whilst the child is agitated. Understanding Palliative factors guides strategy to enable settling. An example is having somebody nearby (e.g. a schoolteacher) whom the child knows, trusts, feels safe with, and is able to talk to the child in a calm and caring manner. The goal is to calm down in safety before any consideration of the behaviour itself.

Practice tip: Build the child's voice

Maximizing communication skills of the child with developmental disability is an essential part of reducing problem behaviours, particularly language around what they feel and what they want.

Initial priorities

Behaviour problems are often multifactorial in cause, manifestation, and required management such that it is not possible to address all aspects at once. In this situation, initial management should address what is important, what can be done easily, and what is most likely to work.

1. What are the child's priorities? For a child with severe disability, this can be inferred from situations most likely to cause behaviour problems and/or distress.

2. What are the parents' priorities? These may include safety of the child, capacity to hold down a job, and care for the child's siblings.

3. What are the priorities of other agencies? Schools, for example, may prioritize the safety of other children and teaching staff.

4. What does the referring doctor and you as the child's paediatrician consider most important? It may be, for example, that the child is not getting enough sleep.

5. Putting all this together, what do you consider to be most important at this stage?

What can be done quickly, early, easily, that is likely to work?

◆ Managing behaviour problems is more likely to be successful when built on initial successes. Examples include avoiding recurrently problematic situations (e.g. school playgrounds at lunchtime) or challenges (e.g. ceasing, modifying or reducing homework). Simple practical strategies may help, such as a trial of earmuffs/noise-cancelling headphones for a child with autism who has meltdowns in loud environments.

Who will undertake management?

The question of what is done by the paediatrician is an individual decision. Some doctors may become deeply involved in behaviour management strategy and therapeutic work with the child and family. Others elect to refer this work to others. For all strategies it is valuable for the paediatrician to remain active in the evaluation of outcomes and the overview of care (see Case management section).

Referring to other providers

Management of child behaviour problems is generally a multi-person activity. Whilst much of the day-to-day work may be undertaken by parents and school staff, other professionals are involved in guiding these staff as well as direct work with the child.

Before any referral is undertaken, it is important to determine whether the child and family are ready and likely to benefit. For families this includes flexibility, willingness to self-reflect, capacity to work together and capacity for change. For children this may include consideration of what they want, desire to help themselves, accept ownership where appropriate, and the capacity to understand and put strategies into practice effectively and sustainably. Work with the child (e.g. stabilizing medical treatment) may be necessary before referral can be effective.

Each paediatrician is likely to have a network of preferred referral providers. In the referral process there is a challenge to communicate referral reasons without telling the professionals how to do their job. It is reasonable and necessary to include information about the background, behaviour, diagnostic formulation, and other strategy in place as well. To avoid telling them how to do their job, communicate an intended purpose (e.g. to help the child learn how to identify and regulate emotional states, or to evaluate cognitive capacity) rather than methodology (e.g. to use CBT or Mindfulness, or to undertake a Wechsler Intelligence Scale for Children, 5th Edition (WISC-V) evaluation).

It is important to clarify roles both initially and on a continuing basis. Is the paediatrician asking for an assessment only or provision of ongoing care? In the case of ongoing care, how should this be organized (e.g. collaboration, take over care)?

If the paediatrician does not have specific referral recommendations, it may be up to parents to find providers. In this case the paediatrician can guide families regarding what to look for (see Further reading)

Practice tip: Preparing parents for successful referral

When you make a direct referral, or when parents find somebody themselves, what should they look for? You can guide them what to look for, what predicts success.

* Parents are easily able to understand what the professionals say to them. Plain language is far better than professional jargon.

* Parents are clear regarding purpose, when and how outcomes are to be evaluated. Purpose should be of demonstrable benefit to the child.

* Parents are clear regarding the strategy, who does what, when, and for how long.

* The therapeutic activity works as much as possible in context—understanding and working with other people (e.g. teachers) and strategy (e.g. medication).

* Families are clear about what is expected of them. The therapeutic strategy involves 'train the trainer' as well as any direct work with the child. This means strategy that builds family understanding and capacity (empowerment).

- The methodology used by the therapist has a sound evidence base.

- The professional will work respectfully in collaboration with the paediatrician, including regular communication of outcomes as well as activities. An example is the use of medication being explicitly integrated with non-medical strategy (medicine as an enabler – see below).

Measuring outcomes

It is just as important to measure behavioural outcomes as it is to measure parameters of change in general medicine. A paediatrician would not manage a child's treatment for diabetes without measuring HbA1c, urinary ketones, and blood sugar level. Information such as 'I think his behaviour is getting better' is not sufficient. Management is more likely to be successful with a valid, objective methodology for monitoring behaviour.

Further reading: Conflicting views of responses to a treatment

Conflicting information may arise because:

- The child's behaviour is different in the presence of different observers.

- People vary in the accuracy of their memory, and recollection may be inaccurate. It may be subject to bias (e.g. saliency bias, recency bias).

- Some observers may have an 'agenda' in reporting behaviour. For example, separated parents in dispute may claim behaviour is worse when the child is in the care of the other parent. Teachers may be working towards specific purpose, such as a diagnosis or medical treatment.

- Individuals impose interpretation, such as Illusory Correlation (1). This is very common and important. People attribute a change in behaviour to some immediately preceding factor, for example a change in medication dose. However, the change in behaviour may have really been caused by any number of other biological or psychosocial factors. When over a period, there have been a number of treatment changes, and a number of intercurrent events, one cannot accurately correlate behavioural outcomes with these treatment changes, especially in retrospect.

Structured approaches to measuring treatment outcomes

The more information to be collected, the more challenging data collection becomes. Limit data collection to what is clearly useful, such as:

1. Changes in the frequency and intensity of behavioural symptoms

2. Level of intended and unintended medication effects

3. Changes in function

The first two of these are essential as regular data. The third can be measured over time.

Data collected at the time of behaviour are also helpful, particularly 'ABC' data (Antecedent, Behaviour, Consequence). Data need to be:

1. **Contemporaneous:** As close to the behaviour as practical. Daily recording is much more accurate than recording progress 6-monthly.

2. **Prospective:** Data collected as it happens is much more accurate than retrospective data.

3. **Regular, at every interval:** For regular data (e.g. daily) there must be a daily entry. If the problem did not occur, then a zero must be recorded rather than a blank. A blank entry creates an uncertainty as to whether there was really no behaviour problem or the reporter merely forgot to make an entry.

Compliance with data collection

Data collection does not come naturally for many families, and compliance is a challenge. The child's behaviour may be overwhelming, taking up their time and energy. The rate of progress may be slow, so the records may seem 'the same' every day.

Some parents (and teachers) may consider they know what causes the child's behaviour and what is likely to work. As a result, they provide interpreted data rather than objective reports. An example is the proposition that 'this medication is no longer working'. The following steps may maximize compliance:

1. Be very clear **why** this data is necessary. Without it, the paediatrician is unable to do their job (e.g. monitoring medication efficacy), making them unable to help their child effectively. Explain that regular data collection is just as important as regular treatment administration.

2. **Data collection that is straightforward.** The methodology needs to be clear and easy. Provide forms to structure the data you want.

3. **Data usage that is clear.** Review progress regularly, with clear expectations that you will look at the information to determine progress and ongoing strategy.

4. **Data collected is important to success.** When they provide the data, spend time looking at and commenting on the information given. Use it to comment on success to date and to set goals for the next review. This allows families to feel their effort has been useful.

A structured, evidence-based data collection methodology, the Developmental Behavioural Checklist Monitoring Version (DBC-M) (2) is presented in **Appendix 5.1** at the end of this chapter. This is based on the work of one of us (Professor Einfeld). It is specifically designed to be easy for parents to collect and record data over an extended period.

> ## Practice tip: Assessment of outcomes drives success
>
> The more specific the intended outcome and its evaluation methodology, the more likely it is that intervention will be successful. People work towards a clear vision of measurable success. Furthermore, as families experience success, they gain confidence for future behaviour management.

Case management

In addition to intervention (provided, recommended, referred) and review of related outcomes, we strongly recommend the role of the paediatrician extends to include coordination and overview. This is particularly so if the prescription of psychotropic medication is involved. For the current episode of behaviour problems, the paediatrician can promote success through activities that build efficacy within the system of care. This is discussed in the section The child's network.

Positive Behaviour Support (PBS)

Paediatricians will often hear that their patients are engaged in, or need to be engaged in, Positive Behaviour Support (PBS). Paediatricians need to know about PBS for two reasons:

1. To apply the principles of PBS in the recommendations they make as part of their practice; and

2. To understand PBS to a degree that enables them to evaluate PBS plans developed and undertaken by others.

PBS developed in psychology as a reaction to behaviourism (3). It is seen by many as a more ethical approach. PBS expands behaviourism to consider four elements:

1. **Understand the behaviour:** Rather than note the behaviour then modify it, ask first what the presumed cause is. From the child's perspective, why do they do this?

2. **Consider context:** An emphasis in PBS is consideration of how the environment may be provoking the behaviour. Interventions should have contextual (social, cultural) validity and remain child centred. An example is to ensure that a behavioural strategy at school can be implemented effectively and safely in that environment.

3. **Build child competencies and capacity:** Behavioural rewards should encourage the development of new adaptive skills rather than just focus on reduction of behaviour problems. The intention is that the next time the child is faced with the same predicament, they have learned a new, more adaptive way of responding.

4. **Promote child well-being and quality of life:** Behavioural interventions should not just be focussed on reduction of a behaviour which is problematic for others but seek to enhance the individual's quality of life more generally.

For more information see the Association for Positive Behaviour Support website.[1]

Working with the child

Reward-based interventions

Common to reward- and disincentive-based behavioural strategy is that understanding of purpose by the child is **not** generally required for for success. Reward strategies to influence behaviour are a universal part of our lives. With children, rewards are regularly used. Yet the paediatrician commonly hears that star charts or other reward-based methodologies have been tried and either didn't work or stopped working after a period of time.

---

[1] Association for Positive Behaviour Support. Published 2024. Accessed June 2025. https://www.apbs.org/pbs.

In response to the comment 'we tried a reward program, and it didn't work', the following conversation, or some variation on this, is common in our experience:

DOCTOR: *'Did Sammy understand what he had to do to get the reward?'*

PARENTS: *'Yes. He knew all right.'*

DOCTOR: *'Sammy, what did you have to do to get the reward?'*

SAMMY: *'Be good.'*

DOCTOR: *'What did you have to do to be good?'*

SAMMY: *'I don't know.'*

Reward strategies are unlikely to work if:

- The parents are not committed.

- The programme is unclear or implemented inconsistently. The time gap from behaviour to reward may be too great.

- The child's developmental age is too low to understand the reward linkage to expected behaviour. This is true, for example, when the child has a mental age below 15 months.

- The child truly does not care about any reward. This is uncommon. It is seen in some very antisocial (usually severely abused) children.

For more detailed information on behavioural strategies and techniques in children with developmental disabilities, see Emerson and Einfeld (4).

> ## Practice tip: Problem solve failed strategy don't just begin other approaches
>
> If parents say they've tried reward strategies and they 'don't work', it's usually because one or more of the seven steps outlined in Table 5.1 have not been implemented properly.

Differential reinforcement

A variation on this standard reward strategy is to facilitate, then reward the preferred behaviour. An example of this would be where a child who is self-biting is given a valued reward when they bite a soft object instead of themselves. This is called either Differential Reinforcement of Alternative Behaviours (DRA) or Differential Reinforcement of Other Behaviours (DRO).

Boundaries, disincentive- and punishment-based consequences

In child development generally and behaviour management specifically, it is important to set boundaries such that children know what is and is not acceptable. This may be for safety purposes only (e.g. keeping the child off the road) or as part of learning (e.g. road safety).

In doing so, the seven steps outlined in Table 5.1 are relevant to how effective these boundaries are. Consequences need to be clear and effective, linked in time, and above all, experienced by the child as a 'natural justice' consequence rather than fear of hurt. Strategy is necessarily adjusted to the child's developmental capacities (e.g. language, memory, comprehension).

There are major differences between aversive-, disincentive-, and punishment-based consequences compared with incentive- and reward-based strategies. First, aversive strategies are based on fear and potential harm (punishment, consequences the child will not like). The child makes behavioural decisions in the context of distress rather than desire, so the intended outcome is necessarily associated with negative emotions. Distress and fear disrupt children's capacity to understand the situation. In addition to compromising any behavioural learning, this is just harmful to the child.

The second difference is that punishment is not easy to construct in proportion to the intended behaviour. It can easily become excessive (e.g. loss of a weekend trip for a small behaviour), even abusive (5). Whilst legislative responses to corporal punishment vary within and between countries (6), some, such as New Zealand, have outlawed corporal punishment primarily for this reason (7).

Finally, disincentive-, punishment-, and other aversive-based consequences just do not work as well as reward-based consequences (8). This has been shown as a consistent finding from multiple studies across multiple contexts. Furthermore, they increased risk of mental health and behavioural problems in later life (9).

It is an important role for paediatricians to help parents manage fair and effective boundary setting whilst avoiding the risks and practices of ineffective and potentially harmful aversive punishment based behavioural strategy. Finding this balance is particularly difficult with children who have disability and behaviour problems.

Table 5.1 Seven steps to a successful reward intervention

Action	Notes
1. **Who**: Engage all the key players in the child's life in the reward programme, to the greatest extent possible.	The child should see that both parents are participating in the planning and delivery. Where appropriate, have the same target behaviour and strategies at home and at school
2. **What**: Address one behaviour at a time, usually tackling first the behaviour which is causing the most concern.	The parents decide what the target behaviour will be, not the child.
3. **Clarity**: The behaviour must be easy to understand by the child and the parent and described in specific not general terms.	Clarity of behavioural expectation, including precision as to whether the behaviour has or has not occurred. Examples: Clear instruction ◆ Do not hit or kick your sister Unclear instructions ◆ Do what you're told ◆ Be respectful/good
4. **Time**: The time interval between behaviour and reward has to be close enough to be within the child's time concept.	◆ Children whose mental age is young may need the reward twice daily or more. ◆ It is no good offering a reward at the end of the week if the child doesn't have a concept of what a week means. ◆ Star charts are a means of giving an interim symbolic reward (the star) towards the substantive reward at a later time after an agreed number of stars.
5. **Motivation**: Pick a reward that matters to the child.	◆ The reward should be such that if the child doesn't get the reward, it is a big loss to them. ◆ The child should participate in the decision about the reward with their parents. ◆ The reward may need to change over time. ◆ The size/value of the reward should reflect the degree of effort you are asking of the child and be sustainable.
6. **Use reward to build capacity**: Try to teach and reward a more adaptive way of managing the problem situation.	◆ The reward programme should enhance skills if possible.

(*Continued*)

Table 5.1   Continued

Action	Notes
7. **Review before proceeding:** Check that the child can describe the reward programme to you.	Ask the child to say: ◆ What they need to do/not do ◆ The reward they will get if this occurs ◆ When and how they will get the rewards Parents should be confident they can undertake and sustain the strategy.

The following considerations are based on the Policy Statement of the American Academy of Pediatrics: Effective Discipline to Raise Healthy Children (10):

1. Prevention (anticipatory guidance) is better than managing problems after they have occurred.

2. Strategy is more effective when pre-considered compared to 'made up' on the spot.

3. At all times, those undertaking behaviour management need to be calm themselves. In the presence of elevated adult emotion, action taken is less likely to work and more likely to be harmful.

4. Consider the purpose. To what extent is it essentially safety (not requiring the child to understand) versus learning? This influences choice of strategy.

5. Intended outcomes of all strategies need to be clear, measured, and reviewed.

6. When managing a 'don't' purpose (e.g. don't hit your sister), always couple this with a 'do' alternative so the child knows what to do instead in the same situation. When they do what has been proposed, this can be reinforced with reward-based strategy.

7. The term 'punishment' implies children had full understanding and choice prior to the behaviour. This is not usually the case with problem behaviours of children with disabilities. Punishment is a punitive consequence rather than an optimized strategy for behavioural learning. It should be avoided.

Physical restraint

Physical restraint is a particular form of aversive behaviour management. By definition it is against the child's wishes. It is an action rather than the threat of an action (punishment). For this reason, physical restraint is often considered as an ethical, human rights issue.

Restraint is necessary in some circumstances, for example the child who does not understand road safety and is at risk of running onto the road. Restraint is necessary to hold children still for medical procedures (e.g. lumbar puncture), and for the immediate management of dangerous agitation and aggression, for example in the emergency rooms.

Physical restraint (e.g. holding a child still) and social exclusion (putting a child in a room by themselves) are recurrent challenges in the behaviour management of all children, particularly those with disability. It is a short-term measure to **manage a situation,** *not* a successful strategy for sustained behaviour change. The following guiding values and principles are based on guidelines for health (11) and educational (12) services:

1. The child's experience should always be considered. To what extent do they understand what is going on? To what extent does it generate fear for the child?

2. Those undertaking physical restraint must remain calm and objective. Anger and fear are likely to be picked up by the child with the likelihood of worsening the situation.

3. When used, it is a short term tactic used only to defuse and manage an otherwise dangerous situation.

4. When used, it should always be followed by behavioural analysis and planning (as outlined in this book) towards the goals of prevention and more effective behaviour management.

5. Consideration and use of physical restraint, particularly at an institutional level (such as schools) should be undertaken within an ethics- and values-based system so that practices are reviewed and accountable to independent standards.

Cognitive behavioural interventions

Behavioural strategies can be combined with methodologies that build on a child's understanding of themselves, utilizing their desire to help themselves. Two such common strategic approaches are Cognitive Behavioural- and Mindfulness/Acceptance-based therapies. There is overlap between these.

Cognitive approaches are based on the understanding that behaviour is not only influenced by mood, motivation, and perceived rewards but also by cognition (thoughts, beliefs, and attitudes). Cognitive therapy attempts to build awareness of dysfunctional beliefs, examples of which include:

◆ **Catastrophizing:** A relatively minor adverse experience is automatically regarded as 'the end of the world'.

◆ **Overgeneralization:** Because that child doesn't like me, no-one likes me.

- **Excessive self-blame:** Not seeing that other factors contribute to a problem as well as one's own shortcomings.

- **Discounting the positive:** Only seeing the negative side.

- **Disproportion:** Excessive estimates of threat or risk.

- **Disproportionate responsibility:** Excessive 'should' or 'ought' thinking. For example, the child feels they should be able to meet a parent's expectations, even if unrealistic.

Successful CBT has several prerequisites. First, the child or adolescent needs the capacity to develop sufficient insight into their own thought processes. This generally requires the maturity and intellectual capacity of a typical school-aged child, although suitability is a clinical judgement.

Second, the child or adolescent needs the willingness and capacity to 'own' their problem to a sufficient degree, with a desire to understand and help themselves, and a capacity to sustain the necessary effort.

Finally, the child or adolescent needs the stability of function (mood, attention control, life circumstances) necessary sustain implementation of strategy.

Change is more difficult when patterns of dysfunctional thought have been present for some time and have become embedded. When a child's thought patterns are well entrenched or very dysfunctional, professional support requires both expertise and the opportunity to provide the necessary frequency of intervention (e.g. weekly sessions). In these cases, it is usually necessary to refer to a psychologist for their expertise and service capacity.

The simultaneous use of medication may be appropriate, in order to 'enable' therapy optimally by temporarily lowering the child's load of anxiety or distractibility. It is uncommon that paediatricians would provide CBT themselves. However it is sometimes possible to utilize some of the strategies on an informal basis, particularly after becoming aware of the child's dysfunctional thinking.

Further reading: Stages of CBT

1. Making the child aware of their dysfunctional thinking in the context of situations (usually some form of threat) and the behaviours the child undertakes in these situations. This is a careful process so the child understands and accepts rather than feels foolish or blamed.

2. When the child is calm, examining what is the 'scientific' truth that still holds in these situations. This may involve exploring a number of alternative interpretations, then choosing what is most likely to be correct. This has to be the child's choice.

3. Practising offline: noticing the dysfunctional thoughts and directing attention to thoughts they have chosen as likely to be correct. This is a conscious, effortful, and psychologically challenging process as the child may feel less safe if they let go of the dysfunctional thoughts that have served a purpose up to this time.

4. Strategies to energize, evaluate, and reward implementing alternative responses in real-time, real situations. This would involve review by the paediatrician to problem solve and provide motivation.

Mindfulness, acceptance, and commitment-based strategy

Mindfulness, acceptance, and commitment methods have deep histories, for example within Buddhist tradition. They potentially extend the clinical benefits of cognitive behavioural strategy. A valuable property of these strategies is that they identify and build upon what already exists and motivates. They enable each child (adolescent, adult) to be active participants in decision-making from the outset.

As with CBT, mindfulness requires capacity on behalf of the child to understand, along with some desire to help themselves.

Appendix 5.2 elaborates a series of steps adapting mindfulness, acceptance, and commitment to the challenge of child behaviour problems that the paediatrician can adopt in practice. The same sequence of considerations is useful in helping parents reconcile difficult challenges in their personal journey of parenting children with disability.

Working with the family

Potential for blame

Addressing family matters can be uncomfortable in paediatric practice where the general assumption is that parents act in the best interests of their children. Parents may feel blamed, that their parenting is the cause of the child's behaviour problems. The following approaches are helpful:

1. Explicitly recognize that parents care. They have sought help for their child.

2. Emphasize their importance, noting what they have already achieved. Parenting approaches are sound but there is more they can learn.

3. Listen, understand, and appreciate the difficulty they experience managing their child, along with any inadequacy, shame, or guilt they may feel. It is likely they are doing their best under the circumstances.

4. As the child has a developmental disorder, as parents they cannot be expected to know everything about it. This includes behaviour as well as function. Learning additional skills is necessary to be effective parents, just as it is with conditions such as diabetes.

5. Improved skills have general benefits for everybody, including themselves as parents as well as siblings.

6. Skills are practical and not too difficult to learn. With practice they become easier.

Separated parents

Managing behaviour problems requires sustained, consistent, and coordinated parent strategy over time. This is more difficult when parents are separated, or when parents are together but not collaborative.

A more severe problem is where one parent recruits the child to actively, even intentionally undermine the status and role of the other parent (parental alienation). This has been considered a form of child abuse (13), given the severity of consequences it has for children. This may be more common when children have a disability, where one parent insists that only they understand the child and know how to manage.

A common challenge is parents who have shared decision-making responsibility but are unable to agree, making it impossible for an intervention strategy to be undertaken. Sometimes a legal resolution to this impasse is needed before ongoing paediatric management can be undertaken successfully.

A clear methodological agreement is needed. This begins by engaging all stakeholders in a clear arrangement. For more information on this see Chapter 3 (Assessment) and the Further reading below. It is best to establish ground rules from the outset that are explicitly stated and revisited as needed. Examples include no aggressive behaviour and an agreement to stay in the session until the end. To assist talking to separated parents, see Further reading in this chapter regarding multidirectional partiality, circular questioning, and strategies to encourage perspective taking (seeing the world as other family members see it).

Further reading: Working with separated parents

When working with medical conditions, such as diabetes, there is a central core of scientific objectivity (e.g. HbA1c) that helps align parents. When working with child disability, there may be greater disagreement between parents due to differences of beliefs regarding nature, severity, causation, and management. These differences are commonly amplified when parents are in conflict. Here are some practical tips. They apply from the outset, assessment, and particularly ongoing care.

Clear arrangements

1. **Prepare** for challenges before they arise. Situations and issues that may be sources of conflict include:

   ○ Booking and notification of upcoming appointments (e.g. who do SMS reminders go to).

   ○ The rights of each parent to attend appointments (e.g. when a parent unexpectedly turns up).

   ○ The rights of each parent to copies of your clinical correspondence, and how each parent receives these.

   ○ Information and beliefs about the child (e.g. 'he is not a problem at my place').

   ○ How decisions are made (e.g. prescribing and taking medication).

   ○ Cooperation regarding medical and non-medical interventions.

2. **Work within the law.** Understand the law as it applies locally. What are the default rights of each parent? Do parents have 'orders' as the outcome of a legal process. How do these apply to individual paediatric practice? If there is ambiguity on specific questions (e.g. right to know of upcoming appointments, medical decision making), seek a legal opinion before agreeing to manage the case.

3. **Your communications.** Based on your understanding of the law and the individual circumstances, be clear about how you will communicate as part of your ongoing clinical care—to whom information is provided, how you expect information to be shared between parents, how sessions are booked, how medical decisions (e.g. medication prescription and usage) are to be managed, and so on. It is recommended that you have a written

policy on communication and decision that covers default situations. In situations where this policy varies due to individual circumstances, it may help to document exactly how you agree to work with the parents

4. **Minimum requirements.** Be clear about what you need in order to provide your service. This may include frequency of visits, how interventions are to be undertaken across households, how communication occurs with school, and so on. If they cannot agree to your terms regarding clinical care, it may not be appropriate for you to provide care, as you are not able to do your job successfully.

5. **Boundaries.** Be clear what you will not do. An example may be hiding information of importance about the child from the other parent or colluding with what the other parent is told.

6. **Exit conditions.** In situations where parents cannot agree on basic medical decisions (e.g. use of medication), it may be appropriate to identify that you cannot work successfully towards the child's well-being and suggest legal resolution of the impasse.

Communicating clinical information

1. **Objective data and sources of information.** It is essential to differentiate the behaviour reported by a parent from behaviour observed directly by the paediatrician. For example, don't write 'the father was abusive towards the child' when the reality is that 'mother stated that father was abusive towards the child'

2. **Clear presumptions.** Be explicit about the child's problems, impairments, and needs as you understand them. These are the assumptions from which you work with both parents. This minimizes arguments about the nature and severity of the child's issues that otherwise may arise, particularly when custody and support is contested.

3. **Pay attention to communication and records.** Be clear, particularly in written communication or any other form that is recorded (texts, emails), regarding purpose. If information is to inform the court, then that is more effective if the purpose is clearly identified. Even when information is for clinical purposes, consider the extent to which it may be used in legal disputes. When in doubt, assume every piece of recorded information may be required in a legal dispute process.

Parent training

Parent training seeks to address parent practices that promote and perpetuate behaviour problems. An example is coercive parenting, associated with conduct disturbances in children. According to Sanders, author of the Triple P parenting programme (14), the goals of parent training are to:

1. enhance the knowledge, skills, confidence, self-sufficiency, and resourcefulness of parents of pre-adolescent children;

2. promote nurturing, safe, engaging, non-violent, and low-conflict environments for children;

3. promote children's social, emotional, language, intellectual, and behavioural competencies through positive parenting practices.

A considerable evidence base has developed documenting the effectiveness of parenting programmes in improving child behaviour and parental confidence and well-being (15). A number of specific programmes have shown effectiveness in parent training. In addition to Triple-P,[2] these include The Incredible Years[3] and Parent–Child Interaction Therapy.[4] Stepping Stones Triple P (16) is an adaptation of the Triple P programme for parents of children with disabilities. It has shown effectiveness in studies of children with ID, autism, and cerebral palsy.

Family therapy

Where apparent family dysfunction appears entrenched and a significant contribution to the child's behaviour, consider family therapy.

In Chapter 2, patterns of family dysfunction which can impede functional behaviour within a family were discussed. Chapter 3 (Assessment) described approaches to family interviewing. As with all areas where specialized skills may be needed, the paediatrician should consider whether to undertake family interventions themselves or whether they should refer. Referral is appropriate when there is family dysfunction but the nature of this is not clear, when an initial set of sessions proves insufficient, or just when time is not available. This can be slow, often difficult work. Addressing this in paediatric clinical practice may be considered family counselling rather than more formal professional methodologies of family therapy.

---

[2] Triple-P https://www.triplep.net/. Published 2015, accessed July 2025.

[3] The Incredible Years. https://incredibleyears.com/. Published 2023, accessed July 2025.

[4] Parent–Child Interaction Therapy. https://www.pcit.org/. Published 2022, accessed July 2025.

Family counselling is most successful when families agree to participate, to attend the meetings, and to work on issues raised for the benefit of their child. It is unlikely to work when one parent participates but the other is 'too busy' or otherwise disengaged.

We repeat the table from Chapter 2 with two further columns: who should participate and a strategy for addressing the problem. It is usual that the strategy will develop or change as therapy progresses. These should be considered ideas or guiding principles to be adapted according to individual needs. This modified table is presented in Table 5.2.

Table 5.2 Problematic family adaptations to disability and suggested strategies

Family Issue	Consequence for Parenting	Who should participate	Strategy
Excessive guilt about the child's disability	Difficulty setting appropriate limits.	Both parents	• Ask parents their views about cause, attributions. • Empathize with their view even if you disagree. • Directly explain the medical cause of disability. Don't assume this has been done before. This can be discussed as a working hypothesis in situations where aetiology is unclear. It is important to have a clear and shared understanding of which aspects of the problem are biologically based and not due to child intention or parental behaviour. This may include some explanation of timing (e.g. 1st trimester origins) as well as possible mechanisms.
Denial of disability	Unreasonable expectations on the child to perform normally.	Both parents	This is usually an expression of unresolved grief. Invite parents to give their views about their child's problems. Diplomatically ask what it would mean for them if their child were disabled and if appropriate, acknowledge the pain of accepting it.

Table 5.2 Continued

Family Issue	Consequence for Parenting	Who should participate	Strategy
Chronic sadness	Lack of opportunity for family to have enjoyment.	Whole family and/or some members	This is likely also to be a stage of grief that may be recurrent or unresolved. Invite parents to retell their story and share their feelings about it. It's OK for them to cry.
Denial of the incurability of the child's problem	Never-ending quest to fix the child.	Both parents	This may be unresolved grief, guilt, or an unnecessarily pessimistic view of the potential quality of life of the child. Empathize with the pain of accepting the child's disability, consider what good quality of life may be for their child in the future.
Marked discrepancy between parents' attitudes to the disability	Conflicting responses to child needs.	Both parents	Ask each to describe their view to you in the others' presence. Invite each to comment on the perspective of the other in a compassionate way, then support them to find some common ground.
Marked discrepancy between parents' attitude to the behaviour (often worse with separated parents)	Ineffectual behavioural rules.	Both parents	Make the consequences of different behavioural rules explicit to both parents. Invite both parents to consider the experience of the child moving across different households. Try to find some aspect of the child's behaviour the parents can agree on that needs to change and suggest a common strategy they can both accept.

(Continued)

Table 5.2   Continued

Family Issue	Consequence for Parenting	Who should participate	Strategy
Blame of one parent	Demoralized and disempowered parenting.	Both parents +/– other blaming parties, eg grandparents	Review what each party sees as the causes of the child's behaviour and address mis-attributions. What can they do to support the contribution of the other parent, and the child?
Overwhelmed by the child's disability support needs	Reduced capacity for constructive management of behaviour.	Both parents	Provide permission for fatigue, and the reduction in workload necessary to manage this. It may involve less therapy for the child. This is a long journey, not a sprint.
Shame	Inappropriate punishment of the disabled child. Keeping the child away from social participation.	Both parents	Such beliefs and behaviours may be a cultural issue. To address this, it is useful to engage a case worker with shared cultural understanding.
Survivor guilt in siblings	Siblings feel obliged to compensate in various ways.	Parents and siblings or siblings alone if older	Siblings need factual information about the cause of their sib's disability, particularly that it is not their fault. Give opportunities to share their feelings and thoughts about their sibling. Provide professional permission for each child to have their own needs understood and met, a prerequisite for successfully helping their disabled sibling.

Media technology and family

A child's screen use is commonly an issue to be considered and managed when children with disabilities have challenging behaviour. Use of digital technology (especially screen-based devices) is a family issue, reflecting family values and the efficacy of family systems for setting reasonable limits (17).

Problematic screen use is both a symptom of and cause of problems. The child who is gaming into the night, for example, may be seeking social community or avoiding challenges at school, or this is a response to family disharmony. The child with severe ID and repetitive viewing of favourite videos may be satisfying a sensory need or expressing a restrictive behaviour urge. These background factors need to be addressed where possible

The families who manage this challenge successfully have active policies that are regularly discussed and reviewed. The general principles include:

- Lead by example. Parent media use behaviour is a powerful influence.

- Manage media usage as a whole-of-family issue rather than rules that target individual children.

- As a family, develop rules based on guiding principles and values, such as reasonableness, life balance, risk of possible harm.

- Talk about media usage on a regular basis, reviewing how these rules are going;

- Some rules may be family wide (e.g. devices out of the bedroom after 9 p.m.). Other rules are better based on child development, just as are rules around independent travel, staying out at night, and other responsibilities. For children with developmental disorders, these rules are necessarily adjusted to child capacity, risk, and needs.

- Rules need consequences. The test of an effective rule is that children can turn off their devices in accordance with the agreed rule without undue distress.

- As possible, learn what children are viewing. Watch with them, talk about it. Try to keep screen use in public areas (e.g. dining room) rather than child bedrooms.

There are many websites providing guidance for families,[5,6,7] based on a large body of research on this issue. For children with developmental disorders,

---

[5] Screen time and children: How to guide your child. https://www.mayoclinic.org/healthy-lifestyle/childrens-health/in-depth/screen-time/art-20047952. Published June 2024, accessed July 2025.

[6] Internet Watch Foundation. https://www.iwf.org.uk/. Published 2000, updated 2025, accessed July 2025.

[7] https://www.aacap.org/AACAP/Families_and_Youth/Facts_for_Families/FFF-Guide/Children-And-Watching-TV-054.aspx. Updated June 2025, accessed June 2025.

guidelines require individualized interpretation.[8] If problems are difficult, the assistance of a psychologist with a special interest in this issue or similar professional is likely to be helpful.

Working with schools

Working with schools presents logistic challenges for paediatric practice. When collaboration with schools is successful, however, this can be one of the more effective and enjoyable aspects of clinical work. Working with schools has several goals:

- To develop a shared explanation of behaviour (hypothesis) as the guide rather than a behaviour → response cycle based on behaviourist policy and without deep understanding of causation.

- To build an explanation of behaviour that is developmental in origin rather than behaviourist in essence. Choice theory (18) is a behaviourally based example taught in some schools without clear consideration of the child's developmental level. Consider the child with social and communication skills typical of a child two years younger. The goal is to help educators adapt their development-based pedagogical skills to behavioural strategy.

- To build a network of sustained communication and collaboration that allows families and schools to plan towards positive outcomes as well as respond to problems. Often the communication partnership between families and schools has broken down before meeting with the paediatrician. Where this has not occurred, a strategy introduced early, such as a school case conference, is a pre-emptive intervention.

- To use this communication network to monitor response to behavioural strategy, problem-solving as necessary.

When communicating with schools,

- Listening is more effective than talking. It is unlikely they will hear the wisdom you would like to share until they feel they have been heard.

---

[8] Screen time and children. https://www.sourcekids.com.au/how-to-keep-your-child-with-a-disability-safe-online/. Published 2014, accessed June 2025.

- Respect professional boundaries. Do not tell staff how to be a teacher, just as it annoys you to be told what diagnosis to make or medicine to prescribe.

- Help them find solutions. Strategies they choose are likely to be more effective than the strategy you propose. Even if you have excellent ideas, it may be best to offer them humbly (e.g. you have seen this work in other schools), with the understanding that they would know whether these strategies, for example, are likely to work in their school.

- Schools tend to operate in a short 'time window'. They can quickly forget, distracted by the demands of the day. Keep the central understandings, goals, and strategies in the foreground.

- The personal touch (phone, video, face to face) is significantly more effective than written information (19).

- Respect for the School Principal is central. Principals do not like it when they are bypassed, particularly with issues that may pose risk or have resource implications for the school. No intervention is likely to be successful in a school without the support of the Principal or a teacher delegated by the Principal.

Paediatric work considers each child as an individual. This is not necessarily the case in schools where pedagogy is often built on an assumption of the 'average' child. Some teachers may require explicit permission as well as information to consider and manage children outside standard strategy (e.g. reduction in homework). Diagnostic categories and medically based information help enable this.

Some staff easily and intuitively generate a compassion-based response to information that helps them understand the child. They are usually successful at finding innovative solutions to problems. Other staff may be tired or carry ideas of their own that do not readily change. It is important to listen and understand the perspective of key staff in order to be most effective.

School policy is important for the paediatrician to understand. The school may be obliged to react in a certain way rather than exercise judgement. An example is the child who has pseudo seizures, when calling an ambulance may be mandatory, despite being rewarding for the child. Another example is protocol to manage a child whose behaviour is considered a threat to students or staff.

Further reading—Planning and running a school case conference

School case conferences are powerful acts of healthcare when done well. They provide an effective foundation for ongoing management of behaviour. As well as face to face, these can be effectively undertaken via video technology.

1. **Arrangements** include where, when, who should attend, the time frame, and who will chair the meeting. One model is for the doctor to chair, but the School Principal may choose to take this role if the conference is at the school. Parents (both where possible) should attend.

2. **Agenda.** A brief written agenda helps the school staff know what to expect and helps keep the conversation on track. An agenda addresses the behaviour (from everybody's perspective), assumed causes and intended outcome before strategy.

3. **Terms.** Begin with your 'terms of reference'. These include acknowledgement that you are not an educational professional and are there to learn. Your goal is to help build consensus, understanding, and strategy.

4. **Listen.** The first round of conversation is systematically to ask those in attendance to talk about their role, observations of the child, and their concerns.

5. **Summary of the challenge.** After the round of perspectives, the discussion tends to drift towards intervention strategy. Before this, summarize what has been said regarding the behavioural problem: the situations, nature, severity, frequency, and so on.

6. **Causal hypothesis.** After an agreed summary of the problem, discussion again is likely to tilt towards strategic recommendations. Formally pause this and indicate you would first like to discuss the question of why this behaviour is occurring. Commonly, this question has not often been formally addressed such that there is no common causal explanation across the school staff from which they can work as a unified group. A key question is the degree to which the child has the capacity to behave otherwise and as expected (a behavioural problem), and the degree to which this is an expression of something the child cannot help (a medical/developmental problem). If possible, draw the conversation to an agreed working hypothesis of cause. One danger to avoid is the assumption that if there is a substantial medical contribution, such that the management of this falls outside the school (e.g. medication). School staff remain responsible for school-based care.

7. **Goals and measurement.** Pose the question of purpose, 'If we were to have this meeting again [e.g. in 6 or 12 month]), what would be the evidence of a successful intervention? How would we know the strategies had worked?'

8. **Strategy.** How will these goals be achieved? Who will do what? A specific recommendation regarding medication (see point 5) is that you propose that medication may not be a valid consideration until after the school has successfully addressed the situations that trigger and perpetuate behaviour problems. Schools may be more motivated for change if this is associated with the prospect of medical intervention.

9. **Communication and review.** How will those involved keep in touch? How will problems be reviewed and solved along the way? How will successes be recognized and celebrated?

Working with the child's network

In addition to family, extended family and friends, the child's world may include school, peers, and community organizations such as religious, sporting, or artistic groups. When the multiple participants in the child's world act collaboratively, outcomes for the child are more successful and sustainable. The Further reading box outlines principles of coordination and collaboration, adapted from system theory.[9]

In working with the child's network, a paediatric default is to talk with parents directly and communicate more widely in written form. For some cases this may be sufficient. When it is not, case conferences are recommended, either face to face or by video/telehealth. These can be highly effective clinically when run successfully with a clear intended outcome defined.

It is often valuable to be active in support for those who work with the child: therapists, the school as well as the family. What is expected of them needs to be achievable and sustainable. They are more likely to succeed in their roles if the paediatrician is actively involved, supportive, and appreciative of their work. An example is working with schools to advocate for more funding towards behavioural support.

[9] See e.g. Systems Theory. https://www.sciencedirect.com/topics/psychology/systems-theory. Published 2020, accessed July 2025.

Further reading: A systems approach to managing the child's network

The child's system comprises those who care about the child and/or have a strong connection to the child. This system of people is likely to have the energy and motivation to manage the child beyond the limited capacity of paid professionals. In addition, the system may develop strategies more adapted and innovative than those recommended by individual professionals. The following is a stepwise guide to managing the child's system:

1. **Define the child's world.** This means formally identifying who is in the system, who has a significant influence on the child, who needs to be involved.

2. **Define the scope of the problem.** What is the problem that the system needs to address? This may vary, for example, if behaviours at school differ from behaviours at home.

3. **Build a unified hypothesis/explanation.** How do the different members of the system understand the child's behaviour? What can be done to align this understanding towards greater accuracy and coherence?

4. **Define the goals/purpose.** If strategy works, how and when will those in the system know? What are the salient measures of outcome?

5. **Differential strategy.** What is appropriate for each member of the system to do?

6. **Encourage innovation.** Rather than a prescriptive approach, what ideas do each member of the group have? When they try these ideas, what happens? In systems theory terms, original and innovative ideas can be considered 'emergent properties' of the system. An example is a grandparent who chooses to spend more time with the child in activities they both enjoy.

7. **Facilitate activity and communication.** How will information be communicated between system members? How will they be kept motivated, encouraged, and take pride in what they have achieved?

8. **The child's role.** In the section on Mindfulness, the value of working with the child to find an acceptance and values-based role in their own care was described. Similarly, how is it appropriate for the child to be part of this network of people involved? What role can they take? How can their ideas and feedback be incorporated into system understanding and behaviour?

Pharmacotherapy

A central goal of this book is to replace a reductionist and often ineffective model of medication use (e.g. medication treats behaviour and needs to be changed when behaviour is not rectified) with a safer and more effective approach to psychopharmacology.

> ## Practice tip: The ethics of prescribing
>
> An ethical (beneficence) approach to prescribing is to ask the question: 'To what extent, taking all factors into consideration, are the expected benefits of the treatment likely to exceed the expected harms for this child?'

General considerations

For children with disability, how is psychotropic medication best utilized in the management of behaviour problems? Many authors have proposed systematic approaches. The following are adapted from Einfeld (20)), organized as general considerations, choice, and usage of medication.

1. **Assessment:** The decision to prescribe psychotropic medication should follow a comprehensive assessment of the child's emotional and behavioural disturbance. Such an assessment will include not only descriptions of the behaviour and a comprehensive formulation of contributory factors but also an assessment of the efficacy of all previous modes of treatment. The paediatrician should try to resist 'knee jerk' responses, despite the pressure of crisis presentations.

2. **Developmental age:** Consider the child in the context of their developmental age. A 10-year-old child functioning at the age equivalent of 3 years old is likely to have the impulse and attention control of a 3-year-old. In this case using 10-year-old diagnostic standards for Attention Deficit Hyperactivity Disorder (ADHD) may result in treatment that does not work very well and may cause harm.

3. **Compliance and safety:** Psychotropic medications should not be prescribed without reasonable confidence that the medication will be given reliably and safely, and that at least minimally reliable feedback about the efficacy of the medication can be obtained.

4. **Consent and decision-making:** Proper consideration should be given to the issue of informed consent with adolescents, particularly with respect to legal requirements. Frequently, the paediatrician is required to make an all-or-nothing decision about a person's capacity to consent. In fact, capacity will be quite variable. For example, an adolescent with mild ID may be able to understand that an antipsychotic may make them feel calmer but may not be able to weigh up the advantages of that against the risk of side effects. Similarly, much younger children, to varying degrees, are able to understand the purpose of medication. If children are included in decision-making, understand, and agree, pharmacotherapy is more likely to be effective.

5. **Integration:** The psychotropic treatment needs to be integrated within the set of other concurrent treatments. It is unusual for psychotropic medication alone to be sufficient. This requires good interdisciplinary communication. As noted above, medication is often an 'enabler' rather than stand-alone behaviour treatment.

6. **Clarity:** The precise target symptoms for which psychotropic medication is being prescribed should be stated. In other words, what exactly is it hoped that this medication will treat? It is very difficult to gain reliable information from global impressions such as 'child will be less disruptive' or 'will be more compliant'. Better to use specific descriptions such as 'child will hit others less frequently' or 'the child will settle more quickly when upset'. See Table 5.3.

7. **Outcome evaluation:** Successful prescribing needs to establish a method for reliably and validly documenting changes in the target symptoms during the course of treatment. Such a system is shown in Appendix 5.1. It is best for the prescriber to ask a particular senior carer who will be observing the patient regularly to keep a chart record. It is also useful to have other caregivers completing charts independently, to provide the basic measure of interrater reliability.

8. **Review and revise:** A danger with medication use is 'set and forget'. Discussion of medication adjustments and 'end game' should be considered even before medication is commenced. Otherwise, children may be maintained on medication unnecessarily long after symptoms have resolved, out of fear that the behaviours will recur, even when the patient's circumstances have changed. When target symptoms have been reduced or absent for a reasonable period, an attempt should be made to reduce the dose. Again, reliable and valid measures of the effect of this dosage change should be available.

Table 5.3 Example behavioural targets and what will not change

Biological Hypothesis	Behavioural Target for Medication	What may not change
Impaired impulse control	The component of behaviour that is impulsive in nature	Behaviour that reflects social immaturity or incomprehension
Impaired memory or retrieval of learned information	Change in behaviour when learned information (e.g. behavioural rules) can be brought into consciousness	Behaviour due to lack of understanding
Distraction, inattention	Behaviour from not listening in the first place	Behaviour due to lack of ability to do what is expected
Disproportionate threat response	Thoughts and behaviours driven by the sympathetic/adrenal response to threat situations	Behaviour due to the child's frustration, anger, or other emotional responses appropriate for the situation
Increased arousal leading to reduced emotional resilience (stress/agitation/anxiety/fear/anger)	Behaviours that occur because background emotion is high, leading to situations where small triggers elicit large responses	Behaviour arising due to choice, confusion, or appropriate levels of frustration and anger
Inappropriate/disproportionate mood responses	Behaviours arising from emotional states not clearly appropriate for the situation (e.g. heightened fear, excitability) or changing unexpectedly quickly	Behaviour arising for other reasons (safety, confusion, frustration etc)
Fatigue	Better self-control with good sleep	Behaviour arising for other reasons

Choice of medication

1. **Rules and guides:** Where appropriate, consider local legislative and administrative requirements and guidelines.

2. **Research:** Prescribing should be based on the best science available, but extrapolation from adult data is often needed. Research may inform use of medication to treat conditions (e.g. ADHD) or symptom complexes within conditions (e.g. anxiety in children with Autism Spectrum Disorder (ASD).

3. **Biological hypothesis**: Where such research is not available, it is still possible to select and evaluate medication based on hypothesis of biological mechanism. This hypothesis addresses presumed contributions to problem behaviour such as impairments of thought and behavioural control (e.g. impulse control, executive functions), and/or impairments of emotional regulation (e.g. threat responses, background mood). See Table 5.3.

4. **Risk**: Consider child risks and family capacity. There are children and families where risks of intentional overdose, intermittent, excessive, or otherwise eclectic usage of medication are unacceptable.

5. **Expense**: Some medications are too expensive for some families.

6. **Family history**: In some cases, other family members have experience using medications. As a general guide, medications that have been effective in genetically related family members are more likely to work for the child.

7. **Pharmacology**: How long will it take for the medication to work? How well does the benefit persist when established? What is the likelihood of missing the 'therapeutic window' with too much or too little medication?

Usage

1. **Dosage**: standard dosage recommendations do **not** necessarily apply for children with disabilities. 'Low and slow' initiation regardless of the child's age and size is safest. Half a tablet may work well even for older large individuals, whereas standard doses may quickly be problematic.

2. **Timing and duration**: Medication use can be tailored. This includes which days and situations, and which time periods within each day. The decision is guided by individual medication properties (e.g. time to build up effect, discontinuation duration, and considerations). Longer-acting formulations have the benefit not only of reducing frequency of administration but there is likely to be benefit also from the stability and duration of bio-availability. Use of shorter acting medications on a prn (intermittent, pro re nata) basis may be appropriate for risk situations.

3. **Pharmacology and efficacy**: General principles of pharmacotherapy must be observed; that is, proper attention should be paid to issues of compliance, pharmacokinetics, drug interactions, and side effects.

4. **Side effects**: Whilst most side effects are clear (e.g. appetite, sleep), some may be more subtle. For children with disabilities, these may be difficult to evaluate. When there is an unexplained change in the child (e.g. becoming more subdued, anxious, or prone to anger), time off medication may determine whether these changes may be related.

5. **Reduction and withdrawal**: Withdrawal symptoms appear commonly in children and adolescents with developmental disabilities if long-standing treatments are terminated suddenly. Sustainable reductions are best achieved with small steps over longer periods of time. An example protocol for reducing antipsychotics is a reduction in daily dose of 20% per month.

Hypothesis-informed outcome measures

A common response to medication trials is the feedback that the medication has not worked, or worked insufficiently well. This may reflect an inappropriately broad range of expected effects. Identify behavioural outcomes from the outset that most directly reflect the causal hypothesis. At the same time, identify behaviours that are *not* likely to change.

Concerns about medication

Some parents think a pill will be a panacea. Others view all medications as poisons. The art is to steer both these extremes to a more realistic understanding. Management of this challenge is addressed with clear explanation, purpose, measures of efficacy, and review, as described above. Even with such an explanation, fears may persist.

Overuse

Concern about overuse of psychotropic medication for behaviour in children with disability are common and widespread. There have also been a number of US surveys of psychotropic drug use in children with autism, demonstrating both high use and a trend for this to increase with time. Rosenberg et al. (21) found in 2010 that 35% of children with autism were prescribed psychotropic medication. This figure rose to almost 50% in a 2017 US study (22), of which 20% were antipsychotics.

The UK Royal College of Psychiatrists issued a position paper specifically for paediatrics, recommending a strategy entitled STOMP-STAMP (23, 24). The purpose of this is that children and young people with ID, autism, or both, have access to appropriate medication, but are not prescribed inappropriate medication. This guide is based on NICE (National Institute for Health and Care Excellence) recommendations. Concern regarding overuse generally is motivation to undertake best clinical practice for individual children.

Restrictive practices

When considering behaviour management for children with developmental disabilities, the issue of restrictive practices is always in the background. These include chemical, mechanical, physical, and environmental restraint and seclusion.

In some jurisdictions, there are official systems to approve restraint if they deem it necessary for the safety of the child and/or those around. Restrictive practices do not require understanding or cooperation on behalf of the child and are likely to be against the child's will. Restrictive practices are a temporizing measure whilst a more successful path can be found.

Use of medication to change child behaviour is potentially viewed as chemical restraint. This concept is defined differently in different countries (25). In some countries the definition is built around two central considerations:[10]

1. The purpose of medication use is to alter behaviour; and

2. The use of medication is not for the treatment of a diagnosed condition.

This definition is problematic in child development clinical practice for several reasons:

1. Psychotropic drugs are intended to alter behaviour.

2. Behaviour problems occur in situations where the condition does not include challenging behaviour in the diagnostic criteria. Common examples are ID and ASD. In these cases, medication is not a treatment of the primary condition.

3. There is no valid distinction between 'behaviour problems' and conditions diagnosed as 'mental disorders'.

Addressing concerns

The issue of consent requires particular consideration when considering medication for children who have disabilities. Every effort should be made to explain the reasoning and purpose to the child at their level of potential understanding and their parents. The more the child and family understands and agrees, the less likely the perception of restraint and the more likely they will use the medication as intended.

When not treating a diagnosed condition with a research-based strategy, clarity of presumed biological causation remains important (see Table 5.3). The more this is understood by families, the more they are likely to understand the role of medication in overall care of problem behaviour.

---

[10] Restrictive Practices Guidance Chemical Restraint. https://dcj.nsw.gov.au/serv ice-providers/deliver-disability-services/restrictive-practices-authorisation-portal/ resources/restrictive-practices-guidance-chemical-restraint.html#Introduction1. Published April 2024, accessed July 2025.

Clarity of intended purpose minimizes the potential perception that the purpose of medication is to inhibit and restrain children in order to alter behaviour. Medication is intended to be capacity building, to enable:

- Greater capacity of the child to manage their behaviour in real time;

- Greater stability and reliability of their behavioural self-control, which improves the child's quality of life and self-esteem;

- Greater capacity to learn, to remember in response to behaviour management strategy, and to use learning to sustain changes in behaviour in a manner that benefits the child;

- Greater capacity to learn developmental knowledge and skills more generally (e.g. more advanced social understandings and behaviours).

Specific medication groups

Paediatricians are assumed to have a working knowledge of these medications. The information below is tailored to children who have developmental disorders with associated behavioural problems. For psychotropic medication in children in general, there are several excellent textbooks.[11,12]

Stimulant medications

Stimulants, including short and long-acting forms of both methylphenidate and dexamphetamine, are the most commonly prescribed class of medication for children, particularly those with disability (26). They have been extensively studied regarding use in the short term and across time.

Although recent reviews support safety and efficacy of methylphenidate in treating ADHD in children and adolescents with ID, there is some evidence to suggest a lower response rate compared to children without ID (40–50% vs 70–80% positive response) (16). Children with developmental disabilities are more likely to have problems with co-occurring anxiety, irritability, sleep disturbance, tics, or seizures. Since all of these can potentially increase on stimulants, careful monitoring is needed.

A specific concern has been risk of seizures. Stimulants are commonly thought to lower the threshold for seizures, but several studies have indicated that they can be used safely in children with well-controlled epilepsy (27).

---

[11] Goodman R, Scott, S. *Child and Adolescent Psychiatry*. John Wiley & Sons, 2012.

[12] Riddle, MA, Campo MJ. *Pediatric Psychopharmacology for Primary Care*. 4th ed. American Academy of Pediatrics; 2024.

> ## Practice tip: Consider finding out what is the best medication from the outset
>
> If it is likely the child will be taking stimulant medication for some time, consider a back-to-back trial of methylphenidate and dexamphetamine from the outset. Ask the family to collect a written record of benefit and side effects for each medication at each dose level. This enables choice of the best medication and dose. As the family (and child) make this choice, they are likely to be more invested in the use and benefits of the treatment.

Non-stimulant medications for ADHD symptoms

The two most common non-stimulant classes for ADHD symptom treatment are serotonin-norepinephrine reuptake inhibitors (SNRI) (atomoxetine) and α-adrenergic (clonidine, guanfacine) medications.

Atomoxetine was introduced as a non-stimulant ADHD treatment option. Head-to-head studies with the stimulant medications, however, at best demonstrated equivalence in some areas of effect (28). In Australia, we observed that the early clinical experience amongst colleagues was complicated by a high rate of side effects, which may have been related to rate of dosage increase and high final dosages. Atomoxetine may be considered in the treatment of ADHD symptoms in children with disabilities when:

- Executive function impairments are a prominent target of treatment (more than hyperactivity/impulsivity)

- They have comorbid anxiety

- Trials of stimulant medication do not work sufficiently well, have problematic side effects, or otherwise are not indicated as first line treatment.

Both **guanfacine** and **clonidine** have demonstrated benefit for the symptoms of ADHD, however neither have been shown superior to stimulant medications. They are useful for children with sleep onset disorders, tic disorders and as an adjunct to treatment of ADHD. Both come in a sustained release preparation, depending on local availability. Both medications have common side effects of somnolence, fatigue, bradycardia, and hypotension. Prescription of clonidine should be undertaken with an understanding of family capacity: specifically, that doses will not be omitted or the medication stopped suddenly, as hypertensive reactions can occur, and that the medications will be managed with safety so there is no risk of child overdose.

Antipsychotic medications

Antipsychotic medications are widely used in children and adolescents with developmental disabilities. Concerns about their overuse have been described above. Antipsychotics are used not only for symptoms of psychosis but for their efficacy as major tranquillizers. They are sometimes helpful in conduct disorders, though side effects often limit their utility.

A recent meta-analysis (29) concluded that antipsychotics for children and adolescents with ASD are more efficacious than placebo in reducing stereotypies, hyperactivity, irritability and obsessions, compulsions, and in increasing social communication and global functioning. A further recent meta-analysis found that risperidone and aripiprazole were more effective in reducing irritability in children with autism than lurasidone or placebo (30).

Use of antipsychotic medication may be 'as required' (prn) as well as regular/continuous. PRN administration can be useful prior to exposure to a situation known to be stressful for the child if the consequences of that stress are severe. It may help early in a behavioural outburst. When the behaviour problem is intermittent and predictable, prn may replace regular use entirely. With this approach, side effects of the medications are much reduced compared with daily use.

First-generation antipsychotics tend to cause more extrapyramidal symptoms, while second-generation antipsychotics cause more metabolic side effects. Side effects of antipsychotic medications were assessed in a systematic review by Pillay et al. (31) and include weight gain, high triglyceride and cholesterol levels, extrapyramidal symptoms, and somnolence. Antipsychotic medications increase the risk for type 2 diabetes. A common clinical perception is that aripiprazole causes less weight gain than risperidone, however this is not supported by research (e.g. (32)).

A rare but important complication of antipsychotic medication is neuroleptic malignant syndrome (33). Features are increased creatine phosphokinase (CPK), fever, tachycardia, rigidity, and altered mental status.

Weight gain associated with antipsychotic medication may be reduced by concurrent use of metformin (34, 35). A guide to dosage for children and adolescents (36, 37) is to start with 500 mg daily for 2 weeks, then titrate the dose over 3 to 4 weeks, depending on patient tolerance up to a total daily dose of 1000 mg to 2000 mg as either twice or three times daily. Metformin needs to be continued for at least 6 months for maximum effect.

> # Further reading—antipsychotics
>
> Siegel et al. Practice Parameters for Use in Children with Intellectual Disability (38).
>
> Volmar et al. Practice Parameters for Use in Children with Autism Spectrum Disorder (39).

Antidepressants

Depression is the primary indication for antidepressants. Diagnosis of depression and other mood disorders is discussed in Chapter 6. Children and adolescents who are dysthymic or frequently irritable but do not clearly have major depression may also benefit.

For children with disabilities there is little research on the pharmacological treatment of depression. Consequently, treatment is guided by practice with typically developing children. Published literature recommends utilizing selective serotonin reuptake inhibitors (SSRIs) for depression on a case-by-case basis.

SSRIs have largely supplanted tricyclic antidepressants in the treatment of depression in this population, given the lower level of side effects. We know of no compelling evidence that one SSRI has any greater efficacy than another. Agitation and nausea are the most common adverse side effects, but this is minimized by increasing the dose gradually. As stated above, it is important to start with small doses, and for this reason SSRIs are available in liquid form present advantages in that titration of small doses is possible. Fluoxetine is probably the most widely used of the SSRIs, although it runs the risk of stimulation (see Table 5.4 for common antidepressants and anti-anxiety medication).

SSRI medications can increase suicidal thoughts, though their net effect is to reduce suicidal behaviour because of relief of depression. Parents should be warned about this possible side effect and report it to the prescriber if it occurs. Suicidal thoughts need evaluation and a safety plan put in place if they occur.

All antidepressants take at least 3 weeks, and sometimes 6 weeks to produce any sustained benefit once the minimal effective dose is reached. For clinical convenience as well as theoretical benefits, SSRIs are best taken in the morning.

There are two genetic variants in the population in the enzymes which metabolize SSRIs leading to a division between rapid metabolizers and slow metabolizers. Rapid metabolizers generally need higher doses of SSRI than slow

Table 5.4 Common antidepressant/anti-anxiety medications

Medication	Daily Dose Range	Side-effects and precautions	Half life (approx)	Notes
fluoxetine	1–60 mg	Often stimulating and can impair sleep.	4–16 days	Formulation may be dissolvable, enabling low-dose liquid administration.
sertraline	12.5–200 mg/day	Increase in suicidal ideation but not behaviour; a rare side effect in this group of children	24 hours	Neither stimulating nor sedating
fluvoxamine	50–300 mg	Often sedating	13 hours	Can help insomnia
clomipramine	6.25 mg. Max dose: 3 mg/kg/day or 200 mg/day, whichever is less	Anticholinergic side effects common: constipation, dry mouth, blurred vision	24 hrs	Considered most effective for obsessional anxiety
mirtazapine	3.75–45 mg	Sedation and weight gain are common	30 hours	A tetracyclic. Safer in overdose than tricyclics

metabolizers. These gene variants can be assessed, but in our view this test is unnecessary unless clinical outcomes are unexpected. The results are not always good clinical predictors of necessary dosage for response. A 'low and slow' approach identifies those who respond to lower amounts.

High serum levels of SSRIs lead to serotonergic symptoms. Symptoms can be mild to severe and may include fatality. Signs of mild serotonin excess are excessive sweating, agitation and increased deep tendon reflexes. Sweating is profuse, occurring even in cool surroundings and without exercise. It may be accompanied by nausea. Stopping the SSRI relieves the symptoms in about 12 hours. The SSRI can be restarted at a lower dose.

Mirtazapine is a potent tetracyclic antidepressant. The tetracyclics do not have the anticholinergic side effects of the older tricyclics and are safer in overdose. Mirtazapine is sedating so it needs to be given at night and can assist with insomnia. Smaller doses paradoxically may be more sedating than higher doses. The main side effect of mirtazapine is weight gain. There is evidence of benefit in anxiety reduction in autism with mirtazapine (40).

Anxiolytics

SSRIs are the mainstay of anxiolytic treatment in children with developmental disabilities, however there are few studies specifically in this population. Evidence for their effectiveness relies on data from typically developing children.

Clinical experience indicates they have a role in the treatment of the full range of anxiety problems seen in children with developmental disabilities. Clomipramine, an older tricyclic agent, is considered the most potent in the treatment of Obsessive–Compulsive Disorder.

Moclobemide is sometimes effective for anxiety when SSRIs are not. It has few side effects of note. Moclobemide is not available in the United States. Buspirone is used in the United States but the evidence for its effectiveness in childhood anxiety is minimal. A systematic review did not support its use in autism (41).

The antihistamine hydroxyzine is used in North America to treat anxiety, but there is no research evidence to support it except perhaps as pre-operative sedation.

Benzodiazepine medications may be helpful in reducing anxiety for shorter periods of time. They are commonly used in the treatment of epilepsy. The two main limitations in using benzodiazepines are:

1. Tolerance development occurs rapidly when used regularly. Therefore, they are best used intermittently, maximum of three times weekly.

2. Disinhibition and irritability are potential problems with benzodiazepine use in children with neurological impairments (42). They occur commonly with clonazepam. When a child with developmental disability taking benzodiazepines for epilepsy presents with these symptoms, it is worth asking the patient's neurologist to consider an alternative anticonvulsant.

The SSRIs have been widely used to manage perseverative and repetitive behaviours, including rituals of autism, preoccupations, and self-injurious behaviour. Studies have shown mixed evidence for effectiveness in reducing repetitive and restrictive behaviours (43). In our experience, SSRIs do not reduce spontaneous interest in rituals and preoccupations. Rather, they make it easier for the individual to be diverted from the ritual. This effect has not been specifically examined in studies. It is presumed to occur by reducing the anxiety arising when ritual or compulsion behaviour is restricted.

Mood stabilizers

Typical bipolar illness is not often seen in adolescents. Instability of mood occurs more commonly, particularly in children with disabilities. This manifests as rapid fluctuation between excitement, irritability, and high levels of activity, alternating with withdrawal, loss of interest, and unhappiness. When this pattern is sufficiently problematic, mood stabilizers may be tried. Medications included in this group are lithium, carbamazepine, valproate, and lamotrigine. There have been insufficient trials of any of these in children with developmental disabilities to allow definitive recommendation regarding efficacy (44)

There are a number of older studies of lithium treatment of disruptive behaviour in people with ID. For example, Langee (1990) found that 42% of individuals treated with lithium improved significantly (45). Lithium has also been widely used for impulsive, aggressive behaviour, although evidence for particular efficacy in this presentation is equivocal.

The important side effects of lithium are impairment of renal and thyroid function. Regular monitoring of these is necessary. Hypothyroidism is common in Down syndrome and is presumably a greater risk with lithium. Lithium also worsens acne. Tremors and other movement disorders are more common side-effects in persons with disabilities, so particular care is needed to monitor for the side effects of lithium in this population.

Lithium has a narrow therapeutic window. Serum level has to be monitored frequently till a stable dosage is reached. A serum level between 0.5 and 0.8 mmol/L is safe and effective. Lithium toxicity can occur at serum levels above this. Lithium toxicity can be precipitated by dehydration. Because of these risks, lithium prescription may be best undertaken only by child psychiatrists or paediatricians who are very experienced with its usage.

Carbamazepine has the disadvantage of requiring frequent monitoring of serum level, which SSRIs tend to raise. Valproate can cause liver disease, especially in younger children, and liver function should be monitored in the initial stages of its use. Valproate is teratogenic and occasionally is associated with development of polycystic ovary syndrome. Lamotrigine is generally safe, but skin rashes may occur, and Stevens–Johnson syndrome is a rare effect.

Antilibidinal agents

Inappropriate sexual behaviour of some children and adolescents with developmental disabilities can cause considerable concern. It may lead to social restriction as well as harm to others. Adolescents with intellectual disabilities may have sexual drive but lack the socialization to restrain them from masturbation in inappropriate places, or behaviour that is sexually intrusive for others. Young people with frontal lobe impairments (e.g. more severe Foetal Alcohol Spectrum Disorder (FASD)) may have reduced capacity to regulate sexual drive. Adolescents with autism may have a preoccupation with sexual behaviour which is problematic. Some young people may have forensic proceedings against them because of inappropriate sexual behaviour.

The pharmacological reduction of libido requires ethical consideration. Medication should be used as a last resort in situations where efforts to redirect inappropriate sexual behaviour through contextual change, behavioural and educational means have failed or are unavailable. When medication is used, non-medication strategies should continue as they may become more effective.

Cyproterone is used in this situation. It is active orally, reducing testosterone levels and usually sexual interest. It can be associated with weight gain. It may also delay epiphyseal closure in prepubertal boys. Luteinizing-hormone releasing hormone (LHRH) analogues are the most effective and safest method for reducing testosterone levels over prolonged periods, but they are expensive and of limited availability. In such cases suppression of this natural aspect of human function may be in the best interest of the patient. These issues are discussed in detail by Sajith et al. (46).

Melatonin

Where disturbed sleep and fatigue are associated with difficult child behaviour, correction of these problems is an obvious early step. Whilst melatonin usage may be safe and effective for primary sleep disorders and those associated with developmental disorders (47), good medical practice necessarily considers the full picture of paediatric sleep hygiene.

Continuing care following initial management

The focus of this book has been the assessment, formulation, and management of challenging behaviour in children with diagnosed disability. It would be a mistake, however, to imply that behaviour problems can always be effectively and sustainably managed in every child with a diagnosed developmental disorder.

Unexpected, underachieved, and unachieved outcomes

Outcomes achieved may be insufficient or different from expected. In these situations, it is tempting to change medication and try again. This can lead to a cycle of reactive decisions that may or may not be successful.

If outcomes are not as expected, review the causal formulation. What is the most likely explanation? What changes to the diagnostic formulation are necessary to include the outcomes as they occurred? How does this modified formulation inform future strategy?

Continuing care/anticipatory guidance

For many forms of disability, impairments lead to persisting problem behaviour into adult life. Understanding the likely natural history and associated risk informs how management is best organized into the future. Regular ongoing care enables capacity building towards the best quality of life as an adult. This is the essence of anticipatory guidance.

1. **Children who will need significant levels of care in adult life.** For children with substantial functional disability (e.g. ID, severe ASD), adult life requires supports for daily living. The greater the challenging behaviour during adult life, the greater the workload for these supports. Regular paediatric care enables continued capacity building towards the best adult quality of life. Example goals of care include learning to manage frustration without aggression and more effective settling when upset.

2. **Children who may live independently, but with significant ongoing challenges.** This group includes FASD, ASD, learning disorders, more severe ADHD, Post-Traumatic Stress Disorder, and Attachment Disorders. Individuals may live independently as adults, however the risk of problem behaviour remains strong. Regular ongoing care enables building insight and self-efficacy as well as more effective frustration management.

3. **Children whose behaviour problems may be transient.** For this group, the behavioural episode is an opportunity to course-correct, to learn skills that will benefit them throughout their life. Continuing care is an opportunity to embed these changes.

Walking the journey with the family

For all children, particularly those in the first two groups above, 'walking the journey' with the family through regular consultation sessions is valuable, even necessary. As noted above, this enables thinking about the future and preparing for it as possible.

In situations where problem behaviour persists or changes slowly, the benefit of regular care and support is primarily for the family, through validation, advocacy, and a regular sympathetic ear. Whilst a lack of change in the child's behaviour may be frustrating for the paediatrician, it is our experience that regular support is treasured by families as a cornerstone of their ongoing care.

Chapter summary

This chapter discussed strategies for managing child behaviour problems, organized in sections. The first two sections are applicable to all children:

1. Initial priorities
   - Safety of the child
   - Safety of others
   - Child health

2. Preparation and planning
   - Defining intended and evaluable outcomes from the outset
   - What should be done first (priorities)
   - Managing referrals and professional collaborations
   - Case overview and coordination over time

For individual child situations, choice of strategy will depend both on diagnostic formulation, and what is available to the paediatrician.

1. Non-medication strategies:
   - Non-medication strategy with the child (behavioural, cognitive, and mindfulness-based methods)
   - Working with families (parent training, family therapy). This includes working with families that may be separated or have other challenges.
   - Working with schools
   - Working with the child's community network

2. Psychotropic medication
   - General principles for using medication in the management of child behaviour problems, including valid monitoring of outcomes
   - Specific medication groups

Continuing care is vital as behaviour problems tend to recur in children with developmental disorders. Regular continuing care supports prevention and optimization beyond treatment.

Appendix 5.1—Developmental Behavioural Checklist

Daily Monitoring of Behaviour using the DBC-M

When daily monitoring of specific behaviours is needed, the DBC-M may be used.[13] This allows for up to five behaviours to be scored daily. Using the DBC-M requires far less time than completing the full DBC versions. Thus, while the DBC-P, DBC-T, or DBC-A are recommended for assessment purposes, the DBC-M is often used in clinical interventions with individuals to map progress. For example, a behavioural intervention is introduced to reduce certain disruptive behaviours in an adolescent who has moderate ID. The full DBC-P assessment has noted hitting, running away and biting, and these are deemed to be the most disabling problems.

By following the method described below, the DBC-M can be used to monitor the success of intervention. As only up to five items are being scored daily, the DBC-M can be completed in 1 minute. It is often useful to ask two parties to record the DBC-M blind to each other's scores, for example mother and father or two care workers in a group home. This serves as an informal inter-rater reliability check. Because the DBC-M requires so little effort to complete, it has often been used daily for prolonged periods such as a year or more. This is very useful for assessment of episodic variations in behaviour disturbance, such as disturbance associated with the menstrual cycle or varying with occurrence of epileptic seizures.

How to use the DBC-M

Specifying target behaviours

Specify up to five target behaviours to be recorded. The behaviour descriptions should be specific, for example 'Hits or kicks other people' rather than

---

[13] DBC Information Package. Monash University. http://www.med.monash.edu.au/assets/docs/scs/psychiatry/dbc-info-package.pdf. Published 2004, accessed 2025. Developmental Behavior Checklist 2 (DBC2) ©Western Psychological Services, 2018

'aggressive'. It is best to use items of the DBC-P, DBC-T, or DBC-A where appropriate, as they have been checked for inter-rater reliability. However, you can also create your own behaviour descriptions.

Write the behaviour descriptions on the DBC-M behaviour monitoring chart in the column labelled 'Behaviour'.

Daily behaviour ratings

Record the date for each day of rating in the row labelled 'Date'.

The parent or carer of the person being described should give a daily behaviour rating for each behaviour, using the key 0 = not a problem today, 1 = somewhat of a problem today, 2 = very much of a problem today. Figure 5.1 shows an example of a completed DBC-M Behaviour Monitoring Chart.

Calculate weekly totals for each behaviour

Calculate the weekly totals for each behaviour by summing the numbers across each row and enter the total in the final column of each table. Totals across all behaviours can also be calculated by summing each row.

Creating graphical displays of the trends in target behaviours

By plotting the weekly totals for each behaviour, or for all behaviours combined, it is easier to see trends in the frequency of target behaviours. Create a graph by plotting weeks along the x-axis and weekly behaviour ratings on the y-axis.

Using the DBC-Score to store and graph DBC-M data

The DBC-Score, the scoring software for the Developmental Behaviour Checklist, is a set of spreadsheets designed to score and store DBC data. For the DBC-P, DBC-T, and DBC-M, the DBC-Score produces a printable report for each checklist entered and also stores entered data in a format which can be retrieved at a later date, and can be transferred into statistical analysis programs.

For the DBC-M, the software stores data, including the target behaviours and weekly totals of ratings for each target behaviour. It quickly generates graphs of ratings for each behaviour and for all behaviours combined. The DBC-Score is able to store and graph up to 52 weeks of data for each subject. Stored data can be retrieved at a later date and can be transferred into statistical analysis programs. An example of a graph from the DBC-Score is shown in Figure 5.2.

DBC Monitoring Chart (DBC-M) ©Western Psychological Service 2018															
	0 = not a problem today 1 = somewhat of a problem today/moderate problem 2 = major problem today														
	Date														
Behaviours							Weekly Total							Weekly Total
1.															
2.															
3.															
4.															
5.															
	0 = not a problem today 1 = somewhat of a problem today/moderate problem 2 = major problem today														
	Date														
Behaviours							Weakly Total							Weekly Total
1.															
2.															
3.															
4.															
5.															
	0 = not a problem today 1 = somewhat of a problem today/moderate problem 2 = major problem today														
	Date														
Bahaviours							Weekly Total							Weekly Total
1.															
2.															
3.															
4.															
5.															

Figure 5.1 DBC data collection tool

Week No: 1								
Behaviour	**Date**							**Week Total**
	2Oct	**3Oct**	**4Oct**	**5Octl**	**6Oct**	**7Oct**	**8Oct**	
Hits or Kicks others	2	1	1	2	0	1	2	9
Screams	1	0	0	1	0	0	1	3
Licks objects	2	1	2	2	2	1	2	12
Steals food	0	2	1	2	2	1	0	8
Urinates outside toilet, though trained	0	0	2	0	0	2	0	4

Figure 5.2 Example DBC data

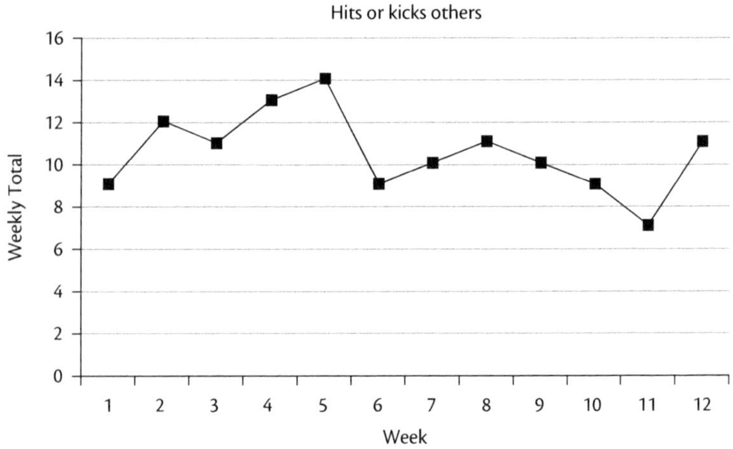

Figure 5.3 Example DBC progress over time

Appendix 5.2—A stepwise mindfulness strategy

Mindfulness, acceptance, and commitment are a powerful set of concepts used to facilitate personal change. They have a deep history. This appendix discusses application of these concepts to work with children who have the capacity and desire to address their behaviour.

This is an approach that can be undertaken successfully in paediatric practice. It can be combined with other strategies, such as the use of medication, with the child's understanding and cooperation.

1. Identify the child's personal values

What are the values a child holds to be important? These values express themselves in behavioural choice when the child is happy, safe, and motivated. They define who the child would like to be, who they enjoy being. Example values a child may identify for themselves include:

- Fairness

- Bravery

- Honesty

- Integrity

- Respect

- Collaboration

- Loyalty

- Caring/compassion

- Effort, persistence

- Creativity, innovation, originality

One approach to eliciting child values is to explore what the child enjoys, what they respect and believe to be important. In the stories that arise within this discussion, a set of values can be elicited and articulated. If they are accurate, the child will generally agree. An example is the child playing team sports. They may value fairness (playing by the rules, everybody equally). They may value effort (playing well, consistency) as well as competency, honesty (if they break the rules), and self-control (not having behavioural responses to referee judgements). They may value the experience of team participation.

2. The issue to be examined

This requires talking about the child's behaviour. If they trust you, feeling safe in the conversation, we recommend you discuss the behaviour problem as if you were watching a video taken when the behaviour occurs. It is important they appreciate this will not be a sophisticated form of blame or judgement, instead a respectful path to helping the child build their capacity and autonomy.

Rather than characterize this behaviour as 'good', 'bad', 'intentional', or some other attribution, consider the extent to which these behaviours deviate from the child's values. As a measure of the behaviour, the less they reflect the child's values, the 'bigger' the problem. Undertaken gently, children hopefully can see that their behaviour is not the expression of the kind of person they wish to be, regardless of the justification they derive from the situation.

3. Agreed explanation

We have reached agreement that the behaviour occurs and does not reflect the child's values. What is the reason for this from the child's perspective? Example possibilities include:

- They were tired, operating out of impulse and instinct rather than with the maturity of their healthy selves;

- They were angry, upset, afraid, and responded out of this emotion, a form of self-defence;

- They were confused, perhaps misinterpreting or failing to think about the experience or intention of others;

- They chose the behaviour as a rational response to the circumstance because it was 'correct', without considering the path to being most 'effective'.

A key to each of these hypotheses is to retain the locus of responsibility and control within the child. If they attribute causation solely to others, for example 'they made me do this', they will not understand and learn how to manage themselves.

The medical perspective on these alternatives is critical. If a child has an exaggerated threat response, the medical perspective is that the child experiences an 8/10 emotional reaction to a situation that, objectively, may be a 3/10 threat. The proposition here is that their brain 'overinterprets' the threat, a biological process that is not their fault, or even under their capacity to choose or moderate. Similar medical-based understandings can be introduced for behaviour that is impulsive (particularly when tired or upset), or fails to pay attention to or understand the other person's true intention and experience.

At the end of this stage, the intended outcome is an agreed hypothesis that has clear and agreed biological presumptions. Tonally this is a scientific analysis, avoiding accusation and critical attribution. The biological presumptions are critical to get out of the loop of concepts such as chosen intention, laziness, malice, or other attributions that perpetuate the situation.

4. Acceptance—intellectual

An understanding and acceptance-based strategy will not work unless they agree with the working explanatory hypothesis. This is not as straightforward as it sounds. A child may be deeply resistant, for example, to any proposition that there is anything 'wrong' with them.

Children (and adults who care for them) may be invested in an existing set of explanations for the child's behaviour. The child may believe, for example, that they can overcome the problem if they just try harder. The parents may believe the child is doing this on purpose.

The first step—defining the child's innate values—helps here. Using values, enquire about intention. It is unlikely the child intends to behave in a manner that does not reflect their values. Enquire about the likelihood that this is an effort deficiency. In reflecting on values, the child may be able to see they are struggling with a biologically based problem rather than just not being good enough in some undefined way. The goal of this acceptance step is a collective agreement about what is going on.

5. Acceptance—emotional

When these conversations are undertaken respectfully and gently, it is common for parents and often children to cry. For parents, this may be a moment of compassion, understanding how difficult it has been for their child, or how harsh they believe they have been. The emotional challenge of acceptance for children is different. Some embrace the explanation, others resist the possibility that there is 'something wrong with them', afraid of the imperfection, vulnerability, or responsibilities that may arise. In our experience, however, embracing a hypothesis is more than intellectual assent. It can be a significant bereavement and emotional adaptation.

6. Personal values—properties of the solution

If the hypothesis is correct, what personal values does the solution reflect? What is meaningful to the child? When children undertake choice-based behaviour that reflects and channels their values, it is more likely to work. What can they look back on, feel proud of? Common values to be incorporated into solutions are:

- **Bravery**—what is the expression of bravery in these situations that is meaningful to the child. An example is the choice to walk away rather than shouting or hitting.

- **Effort**—what can the child do that requires effort but is achievable, sustainable?

- **Fairness**—what does this mean for the child? As they are fair to others, as others are fair with them?

- **Caring**—if they care, can they learn to modify behaviours that may hurt others, physically or verbally?

- **Intelligence**—what are clever ways of managing this challenge?

7. Strategy

With values guiding strategy, what is it possible to actually do? What could they achieve and feel proud of? What can they commit to?

Strategy is most likely to be sustainably successful if it begins with smaller, achievable goals with clear, positive feedback. This may involve:

- Rehearsed verbal propositions to guide the behaviour, such as 'I am upset, and I am going to my room to calm down.'

- Self-talk of change—for example 'I don't want to do that anymore; I want to do this instead.'

- Strategies to seek clarification in situations where misinterpretation of intention is common.

The more a child is involved in the development of strategy, in our experience the more likely it is that the strategy will work. Likewise, the more the micro-steps are recognized and celebrated, the more each stepwise change will be sustained.

8. Commitment and review

This is a team effort. A particularly important aspect is the appreciation of others, particularly parents, of the bravery and effort involved. This is a child with cerebral palsy finishing a race. This is a child with social anxiety talking in front of the class, the child with autism managing their role in a school play. It is hard for the child. If feedback fails to recognize and support in particular the effort and courage, longer-term chances of success diminish.

In this review process, the paediatrician's role is important. Paediatricians have an appreciation of the biological obstacles faced by the child. It is an honour often to see what the child can do with support and understanding. The paediatrician is also an authority figure, and praise from a person in authority is especially meaningful.

Appendix 5.3—Clinical cases

Case 1. Jack

Jack is a boy with FASD. You have discussed your diagnostic formulation with the family. They know that Jack wants to do the right thing and they have not been able to understand why he behaves as he does. They found this formulation framework helpful, the first time that Jack's behaviour has 'made sense' to them.

Discussion

Beyond reduction of the frequency and intensity of Jack's behaviour, what else are you trying to achieve?

Not only is his behaviour harmful in the here and now, it is also the 'canary in the coal-mine', a warning sign of future harm to Jack. Whilst seeking to reduce frequency and intensity of problem behaviour, the paediatrician's goal is to create a situation where Jack feels sufficiently safe, able to meet expectations, and feel positive enough about himself that the risk of future behavioural problems is minimized.

To achieve this, the 'goodness-of-fit' model is useful. Most would have no trouble adapting classrooms and curriculum for a child with motor or vision/hearing deficits. Jack's situation is fundamentally no different. His challenges are just less visible and evident. It is only when Jack feels safe, motivated, and able that he will be able to learn to self-monitor and self-manage more successfully.

Where do you start? What do you consider to be interventions that may make a difference early?

There may be medical issues the paediatrician can address quickly and successfully. Examples include sleep disruption, poor diet, insufficient exercise, and possible sources of pain/discomfort. There may be local risks, such as elevated lead levels.

Early use of medication (ADHD/Anxiety) may act as a 'circuit breaker', enabling Jack to manage himself more successfully. There is a danger, however, that medication will be regarded as a solution that minimizes the need for associated interventions. The goal with ADHD medication is to balance dose and side effects with duration across time periods where he benefits from the assistance. If this is insufficient to assist emotional regulation/threat response, additional medication may be necessary. The choice of agent may include SSRI, atomoxetine, or alpha-adrenergic medications. In Jack's case, it is possible his brain is sensitive to medication, so a cautious 'low-and-slow' approach is strongly recommended. There is no rush, this is a long-term challenge.

Given there may be trials of multiple medications, the paediatrician will need reliable data to judge efficacy. Systematic monitoring of frequency and severity of behaviour problems is needed.

A key early intervention is to take pressure off Jack. This could include advocacy to stop, reduce or change homework, activities that tire him, and curriculum expectations that he cannot manage. Included is a redirection of his energies towards activities he enjoys.

As the paediatrician does this, others may express the opinion that this is wrong, a reward for bad behaviour. In our opinion, this is where medical advocacy is important. Standard homework for a boy like Jack is like standard cross-country running for a boy with Cerebral Palsy.

What direct and indirect strategies would you undertake with Jack himself?

Jack has to grow up with sufficient understanding and capacity that he not only can manage his behaviour but also function in society with resilience and optimal mental health. In our experience, this can benefit from a long-term relationship with a professional who understands and likes Jack, and who is able to spend the time listening to and guiding him.

Non-medical strategies depend on the paediatrician's experience and the availability of services (e.g. psychology) locally. Sets of therapeutic sessions may assist in modifying discrete problems (e.g. learning to be emotionally self-aware and learning how to calm down), however success depends on capacity and motivation on Jack's part.

What direct and indirect strategies would you undertake with Jack's family?

The paediatrician's immediate contribution may be in consideration of a behavioural strategy at home (see Table 5.1). What situations are priority, requiring management? What can be left until later? How are they able to improve the clarity, consistency, and effectiveness of what they do?

It is important that the paediatrician does not imply Jack's behaviour arises from the family's ineffective care. It does not. In fact, the paediatrician's gentle support for Jack's family is likely to be critical for Jack's long-term success. For them, the journey is likely to be unrelentingly hard, particularly as the 'gap' between Jack and his peers widens. As noted above, it may help to spend time considering the consequences of early childhood trauma/abuse/neglect as well as the FASD. Trauma leads to a persisting post-traumatic brain response. Neglect leads to persisting disruption of capacity to trust.

As the paediatrician supports the family, the goal is long-term sustainable care. For this, less may be more, particularly regarding therapeutic interventions. What can the family do to take care of itself?

What strategies would you undertake with Jack's school?

Effective communication and collaboration with the school enables them to understand Jack from a disability perspective, to understand what medication is and is not able to do, and provides opportunity to reflect on effective behavioural strategy.

Collaboration enables establishment of a measurement system that captures change rather than binary conclusions for Jack's behaviour. Change is likely to be a slow process.

Often there is tension between default educational expectations (behaviour, curriculum, participation in activities such as sport) and the needs of the individual child. We encourage the paediatrician to be active in advocacy. Jack is biologically different, just as is a child with epilepsy or anaphylaxis risk. It is a categorical reconsideration requiring categorical changes. In the United States, the Individuals with Disabilities Education Act (IDEA) ensures special education and related services to children with disabilities and establishes procedural safeguards to protect the rights of their parents. In Australia, this level of legal support is unavailable, and the same may be true for other countries. This gives greater responsibility to the professional to be the voice of advocacy for the child.

In some cases, there is insufficient capacity or flexibility at the school. In these cases, it is best to identify these limitations early and consider changing schools.

What can be done to sustain changes achieved into the future?

In medical care, there is an established approach to management of 'chronic' conditions such as Cystic Fibrosis and Insulin-dependent Diabetes. This approach combines the best medical treatment with long-term intended and regular care that emphasizes prevention, optimization, building autonomy and agency. The goal is to ensure children are in the best of possible health when they become adults.

The same is true for Jack. He has a chronic condition. Even if the paediatrician is successful in settling his behaviour down, his broader developmental risk persists. What can the paediatrician do to support Jack through to adult life in the best possible shape (behaviour, function, mental and physical health)? A good starting point is a commitment to seeing them regularly, every 3 to 6 months, for example, indefinitely into the future.

Case 2. Jade

Jade is a 14-year-old girl in her second year of high school. She has a diagnosis of high-functioning ASD made four years earlier. Her behaviour has been worsening across the last 12 months, with angry non-compliant behaviour at home and school avoidance. Your formulation has identified multiple contributing considerations.

Discussion

With Jade, where do you start?

With her intelligence and independence of perspective, Jade needs to be an active participant in her own care. An important early goal is that Jade trusts the paediatrician, feeling respected. This is best achieved by taking the time and listening to her. Her anger is unlikely to settle sufficient for effective management until she has trust and rapport.

If evidence suggests Jade has problems with executive function, an ADHD diagnosis and use of medication may enable greater capacity to manage. This is discussed further below.

Whilst changes are being negotiated, it may be useful to have a defined period of time away from school for safety and rehabilitation purposes. This may require advocacy from the paediatrician to remove these expectations temporarily. This may be included as incentive in a behaviour plan to manage sleep and disruptive behaviour at home.

What strategies would you undertake with Jade, her family and school?

An early goal is to modify behaviour at home. Jade's brother particularly needs to be safe. A family-level safety plan that addresses physical behaviour (e.g. hitting), verbal threat, and interpersonal abuse should also be possible without fundamentally violating Jade's sense of safety. It is likely to deeply annoy her, however, so the 'carrot and stick' of behaviour management needs to be precise. Assistance of a professional may be necessary with the step-by-step process of this. It requires clarity (e.g. what is and is not a behaviour that violates the family safety plan) and consistency (e.g. between parents in how the consequences are administered).

A second home-based goal is to modify her screen usage and sleep cycles. Again, the assistance of a professional with expertise in behaviour management (e.g. psychologist) may be necessary for this. This is an early area where setting boundaries with behaviour management may annoy her considerably but does not violate safety.

Medical intervention to assist these early behavioural goals may include her sleep (e.g. melatonin), her disorganization, and likely anxiety (e.g. atomoxetine, stimulants plus SSRI combinations). Medication is unlikely to alter her behaviour sufficiently but may enable her to manage what is expected of her in a better way and benefit from associated strategy.

When considering and using medication it is important to involve Jade each step of the way. She needs to agree with the hypothesis (e.g. executive dysfunction, anxiety, disordered sleep phase), the goal, the intervention, and be an active participant in the evaluation of success. For a seemingly confident yet frightened girl, this involves a degree of self-reflection and acceptance that is likely to be hard for her. She needs to feel the empowerment of medication rather than a message that medication is a tool to induce her to behave as others wish.

There is work to make school safe for her re-entry before she starts to go back. This is likely to include both curriculum (e.g. assignments, homework, subject load, etc.) as well as social adjustments (protection from bullying, a place where she can be with non-judgemental kindred spirits). This may require several conversations for them to understand her needs and adapt as needed. If the school is unable, an alternative school may be required.

Finally, she needs a re-entry plan. This may be graded. Again, this is likely to need external guidance and planning. It should be success based, with Jade actively involved in the evaluation of this success. The basis is that what is expected is reasonable, balanced with expectations of reasonable effort on her part. It is likely she has a level of shame as she re-engages with school. This needs active management, as the truth for her is that going back to school is likely to require considerable courage.

Jade's behaviour at home needs to settle. She needs to re-engage with regular school participation. Beyond these behavioural goals, what else would you like to achieve?

The longer-term goal is to set up a system that is likely to sustain Jade and help her to thrive. The ingredients of this include agency (Jade's understanding of herself and capacity to advocate for her needs), balanced with a world that is clear, fair, and reasonable for her. All information should be explicit as her capacity to infer is limited. At home this includes clarity of expectation and consequence. At school this is a regular process of review, resetting, and general support for Jade.

Fundamentally, life for her is likely to be hard, particularly at school. For Jade to manage and thrive, she is likely to need a sense of connection somewhere, a 'tribe', a place where she belongs.

The paediatric role in this is important. It involves guiding and supporting as she navigates the journey of teenage life. From the outset, it may help to build a vision of her future, of who she will be as an adult—her vocation, her friends, interests, and so on. If she can engage with this vision, you work towards it, shifting the balance from fixing problems to building an intended and desired future.

Case 3. Alfred

Alfred has Down syndrome and moderate ID. He returns to your clinic for further consultation, accompanied by his mother. You have decided to discontinue the stimulant medication on the presumption that it was contributing to his irritability.

There are no concerns regarding aggressive behaviour, but he continues to be somewhat hyperactive and impulsive. At school he has a fenced environment so safety is not a concern. At home, however, he travels into the community with his mother or other carers. Occasionally, he has absconded briefly. It is hypothesized that his behaviour arises from his impulsivity and a lack of understanding of the concept of safety.

School records indicate that he is meeting his educational goals. He has an IQ of 45, with cognitive and language abilities at around 6 to 7 years age equivalent. He continues to struggle with attention and task persistence. The school is focusing on life skills and intends to enrol him in a pre-vocational curriculum next year. His father continues to provide support to Alfred, and Alfred enjoys his somewhat sporadic visits with his father.

His mother cries as she tells you she is concerned about his safety and asks if medication might help. Alfred, aware of her tears, turns to her, gives her a hug, and says, 'I'm sorry Mummy'. Privately, she says she has not been in good health recently, and she worries about his future if she is unable to care for him.

Discussion

How might a formulation structure inform your management of Alfred?

The role of consistent family support is critical. You acknowledge how his mother's loving support of Alfred has been so consistent over the years and encourage her to seek support regarding her own physical and mental health. It is a hard and relentless journey.

Presuming Alfred struggles with uncertainty, the use of structure and visual supports are likely to be helpful at home, in school, and in the community, with particular attention to precipitating causes, such as changes in routine or unexpected demands.

It is important to address the risk associated with running away. Alfred is impulsive, easily excited and fails to understand danger. In practical terms this could be managed with fencing and careful selection of where he is taken. Funded supports potentially enable somebody with him one to one for risk situations. Non-stimulant medications may be helpful but unlikely to fix the problem. It is wise to avoid using drugs like risperidone, with their attendant metabolic side effects.

You discuss with his mother her concerns for Alfred. What might be contributing to his mother's worries about his safety?

Alfred is doing relatively well, and his successes are testament to the enduring love and support from his mother and teachers, and the goodness of fit with his educational plan. His mother may harbour residual guilt regarding the trauma he experienced in earlier years, and this may make her somewhat overprotective of Alfred. Also, her declining health may make her more anxious about his care in the future. These emotions may be contributing to her current concerns about his safety.

His father's role has become clearer over the years. He is an alcoholic. Alfred witnessed domestic violence in earlier years, and this trauma undoubtedly contributed to his aggressive behaviour. Alfred's father engaged in child and family therapy and learned to be less harsh and coercive with Alfred. He has continued to provide support to Alfred, and Alfred enjoys his somewhat sporadic visits with his father. Importantly, the aggressive and disruptive behaviours of earlier years have essentially resolved. His resilience despite past trauma suggests intrinsic strengths in social cognition in addition to these external supports.

How can you help to establish priorities and set goals for the year ahead? How can you help measure progress towards these goals?

Although he has moderate ID, Alfred has made progress in language and cause-and-effect thinking, and he has shown growing ability to use these capacities to think first before acting impulsively. He continues to be inattentive, distractible, and somewhat impulsive, and the question about medication for ADHD remains. Medical treatment needs careful measurement of intended outcomes to evaluate risk versus benefit.

As the central struggle of aggressive behaviour has settled, current care is focused on several goals. The most immediate is his safety. While validating his mother's concerns, it will be important to reinforce that his more unsafe behaviours (such as absconding) have settled. Practical approaches may include working with him on building specific skills to enhance his safety and encourage his independence.

Other important priorities include setting goals for Alfred's learning of basic academic and life skills, as well as his capacity for self-regulation and recreation. Looking beyond the upcoming year, the goal is to prepare Alfred as much as possible for independent adult life.

References

(1) Matute H, Blanco F, Yarritu I, Díaz-Lago M, Vadillo MA, Barberia I. Illusions of causality: How they bias our everyday thinking and how they could be reduced. *Front Psychol.* 2015;6:888.

(2) Einfeld SL, Tonge BJ. The Developmental Behavior Checklist: The development and validation of an instrument to assess behavioral and emotional disturbance in children and adolescents with mental retardation. *J Autism Dev Disord.* 1995;25(2):81–104.

(3) Hieneman M. Positive behavior support for individuals with behavior challenges. *Behav Anal Pract.* 2015;8(1):101–8.

(4) Emerson E, Einfeld SL. *Challenging Behaviour.* Cambridge University Press; 2011.

(5) Durrant J, Ensom R. Physical punishment of children: Lessons from 20 years of research. *CMAJ Can Med Assoc J.* 2012;184(12):1373–7.

(6) Physical punishment legislation. Australian Institute of Family Studies. Published August 2021. Accessed July 2025. https://aifs.gov.au/resources/resource-sheets/physical-punishment-legislation

(7) Kelly P. Corporal punishment and child maltreatment in New Zealand. *Acta Paediatr* 2011;100(1):14–20.

(8) Glicksman E. Physical discipline is harmful and ineffective. *APA* 2019;50(5):22. https://www.apa.org/monitor/2019/05/physical-discipline

(9) Olson SL, Choe DE, Sameroff AJ. Trajectories of child externalizing problems between ages 3 and 10 years: Contributions of children's early effortful control, theory of mind, and parenting experiences. *Dev Psychopathol.* 2017;29(4):1333–1351.

(10) Sege RD, Siegel BS, Council on Child Abuse and Neglect, Committee on Psychosocial Aspects of Child and Family Health, Flaherty EG, Gavril AR, et al. Effective discipline to raise healthy children. *Pediatrics.* 2018;142(6):e20183112.

(11) Masters KJ, Bellonci C. Practice parameter for the prevention and management of aggressive behavior in child and adolescent psychiatric institutions, with special reference to seclusion and restraint. *J Am Acad Child Adolesc Psychiatry.* 2002;41(2, Supplement):4–25S.

(12) Cramer AM, Barnard-Brak L, Watkins L, Fedewa MP. Teacher experiences of restraint events and school district policies on the use of restraint with children with disabilities. *Behav Disord.* 2024;50(1):3–16.

(13) Isailă OM, Hostiuc S. Medical-legal and psychosocial considerations on parental alienation as a form of child abuse: A brief review. *Healthc Basel Switz.* 2022;10(6):1134.

(14) Sanders MR. Triple P—Positive Parenting Program: Towards an empirically validated multilevel parenting and family support strategy for the prevention of behavior and emotional problems in children. *Clin Child Fam Psychol Rev.* 1999;2(2):71–90.

(15) Anita Thapar, Daniel S. Pine, James F. Leckman, Stephen Scott, Margaret J. Snowling, Eric Taylor. *Rutter's Child and Adolescent Psychiatry.* 6th ed. John Wiley & Sons, Ltd; 10 July 2015. https://www.wiley.com/en-au/Rutter%27s+Child+and+Adolescent+Psychiatry%2C+6th+Edition-p-9781118381960

(16) Tellegen CL, Sanders MR. Stepping Stones Triple P—Positive Parenting Program for children with disability: A systematic review and meta-analysis. *Res Dev Disabil.* 2013 May;34(5):1556–1571.

(17) Poulain T, Meigen C, Kiess W, Vogel M. Media regulation strategies in parents of 4- to 16-year-old children and adolescents: A cross-sectional study. *BMC Public Health.* 2023;23(1):371.

(18) Glasser's choice theory. In: Wikipedia [Internet]. March 2017, Updated January 2025, Accessed July 2025. https://en.wikipedia.org/w/index.php?title=Glasser%27s_choice_theory&oldid=1167148304

(19) O'Keeffe MJ, McDowell M. Bridging the gap between health and education: Words are not enough. *J Paediatr Child Health.* 2004;40(5–6):252–257.

(20) Einfeld S. Guidelines for the use of psychotropic medication in patients with intellectual handicaps. *Aust N Z J Dev Disabil.* 1990;16:71–73.

(21) Rosenberg RE, Mandell DS, Farmer JE, Law JK, Marvin AR, Law PA. Psychotropic medication use among children with autism spectrum disorders enrolled in a national registry, 2007-2008. *J Autism Dev Disord.* 2010;40(3):342–351.

(22) Madden JM, Lakoma MD, Lynch FL, Rusinak D, Owen-Smith AA, Coleman KJ, et al. Psychotropic medication use among insured children with autism spectrum disorder. *J Autism Dev Disord.* 2017;47(1):144–154.

(23) Stop the Over-medication of People with Intellectual Disability, Autism or Both (STOMP) and Supporting Treatment and Appropriate Medication in Paediatrics (STAMP). Royal College of Psychiatrists. (August 2021). Accessed September 2024. https://www.rcpsych.ac.uk/docs/default-source/improving-care/better-mh-policy/position-statements/position-statement-ps0521-stomp-stamp.pdf? sfvrsn=684d09b3_6

(24) Branford D, Gerrard D, Saleem N, Shaw C, Webster A. Stopping over-medication of people with intellectual disability, Autism or both (STOMP) in England part 1—History and background of STOMP. *Adv Ment Health Intellect Disabil.* 2018;13(1):31–40.

(25) Muir-Cochrane E. A wicked problem: Chemical restraint: Towards a definition. *Int J Ment Health Nurs.* 2020;29(6):1272–1274.

(26) Doan T, Ware R, McPherson L, van Dooren K, Bain C, Carrington S, et al. Psychotropic medication use in adolescents with intellectual disability living in the community. *Pharmacoepidemiol Drug Saf.* 2014;23(1):69–76.

(27) Hässler F, Thome J. [Mental retardation and ADHD]. *Z Kinder Jugendpsychiatr Psychother.* 2012;40(2):83–93.

(28) Wu CS, Shang CY, Lin HY, Gau SSF. Differential treatment effects of methylphenidate and atomoxetine on executive functions in children with Attention-Deficit/Hyperactivity Disorder. *J Child Adolesc Psychopharmacol.* 2021;31(3):187–196.

(29) D'Alò GL, De Crescenzo F, Amato L, Cruciani F, Davoli M, Fulceri F, et al. Impact of antipsychotics in children and adolescents with autism spectrum disorder: A systematic review and meta-analysis. *Health Qual Life Outcomes.* 2021;19(1):33.

(30) Fallah MS, Shaikh MR, Neupane B, Rusiecki D, Bennett TA, Beyene J. Atypical antipsychotics for irritability in pediatric autism: A systematic review and network meta-analysis. *J Child Adolesc Psychopharmacol.* 2019;29(3):168–180.

(31) Pillay J, Boylan K, Newton A, Hartling L, Vandermeer B, Nuspl M, et al. Harms of antipsychotics in children and young adults: A systematic review update. *Can J Psychiatry Rev Can Psychiatr.* 2018;63(10):661–678.

(32) Schoemakers RJ, van Kesteren C, van Rosmalen J, Eussen MLJM, Dieleman HG, Beex-Oosterhuis MM. No differences in weight gain between risperidone and aripiprazole in children and adolescents after 12 months. *J Child Adolesc Psychopharmacol.* 2019;29(3):192–196.

(33) Neuhut R, Lindenmayer JP, Silva R. Neuroleptic malignant syndrome in children and adolescents on atypical antipsychotic medication: A *review. J Child Adolesc Psychopharmacol.* 2009;19(4):415–422.

(34) Mansuri Z, Makani R, Trivedi C, Adnan M, Vadukapuram R, Rafael J, et al. The role of metformin in treatment of weight gain associated with atypical antipsychotic treatment in children and adolescents: A systematic review and meta-analysis of randomized controlled trials. *Front Psychiatry.* 2022;13:933570.

(35) Ellul P, Delorme R, Cortese S. Metformin for weight gain associated with second-generation antipsychotics in children and adolescents: A systematic review and meta-analysis. *CNS Drugs*. 2018;32(12):1103–1112.

(36) Soliman A, De Sanctis V, Alaaraj N, Hamed N. The clinical application of metformin in children and adolescents: A short update. *Acta Bio Medica Atenei Parm*. 2020;91(3):e2020086.

(37) Wang DD, Mao YZ, He SM, Chen X. Analysis of time course and dose effect from metformin on body mass index in children and adolescents. *Front Pharmacol [Internet]*. 2021 Apr 26;12:611480. doi:10.3389/fphar.2021.611480. PMID: 33981216; PMCID: PMC8107689.

(38) Siegel M, McGuire K, Veenstra-VanderWeele J, Stratigos K, King B, Bellonci C, et al. Practice parameter for the assessment and treatment of psychiatric disorders in children and adolescents with intellectual disability (intellectual developmental disorder). *J Am Acad Child Adolesc Psychiatry*. 2020;59(4):468–496.

(39) Volkmar F, Siegel M, Woodbury-Smith M, King B, McCracken J, State M. Practice parameter for the assessment and treatment of children and adolescents with autism spectrum disorder. *J Am Acad Child Adolesc Psychiatry*. 2014;53(2):237–257.

(40) McDougle CJ, Thom RP, Ravichandran CT, Palumbo ML, Politte LC, Mullett JE, et al. A randomized double-blind, placebo-controlled pilot trial of mirtazapine for anxiety in children and adolescents with autism spectrum disorder. *Neuropsychopharmacology*. 2022;47(6):1263–1270.

(41) Gupta N, Gupta M, Gandhi R. Buspirone in autism spectrum disorder: A systematic review. *Cureus*. 2022;15(5):e39304.

(42) Kalachnik JE, Hanzel TE, Sevenich R, Harder SR. Benzodiazepine behavioral side effects: review and implications for individuals with mental retardation. *Am J Ment Retard AJMR*. 2002;107(5):376–410.

(43) Volkmar F, Siegel M, Woodbury-Smith M, King B, McCracken J, State M, et al. Practice parameter for the assessment and treatment of children and adolescents with autism spectrum disorder. *J Am Acad Child Adolesc Psychiatry*. 2014;53(2):237–257.

(44) Hirota T, Veenstra-VanderWeele J, Hollander E, Kishi T. Antiepileptic medications in autism spectrum disorder: A systematic review and meta-analysis. *J Autism Dev Disord*. 2014;44(4):948–957.

(45) Langee HR. Retrospective study of lithium use for institutionalized mentally retarded individuals with behavior disorders. *Am J Ment Retard AJMR*. 1990;94(4):448–452.

(46) Sajith SG, Morgan C, Clarke D. Pharmacological management of inappropriate sexual behaviours: A review of its evidence, rationale and scope in relation to men with intellectual disabilities. *J Intellect Disabil Res JIDR*. 2008;52(12):1078–1090.

(47) Esposito S, Laino D, D'Alonzo R, Mencarelli A, Di Genova L, Fattorusso A, et al. Pediatric sleep disturbances and treatment with melatonin. *J Transl Med*. 201912;17(1):77.

6

Syndrome considerations

What does the diagnosis tell you about behaviour?

When a child has a clinical syndrome, there are several potential relationships between the syndrome and behaviour problems. The behaviour may be:

1. **A symptom of the syndrome:** An example is hyperphagia in a child with Prader–Willi syndrome. The behaviour is part of the 'behavioural phenotype' of the syndrome.

2. **A vulnerability associated with the syndrome:** An example is problematic behaviour normal for a child of a younger age in a child with intellectual disability (ID), which is problematic because of the child's size.

3. **A consequence of treatment:** The behaviour may be a consequence of side effects of treatment of the syndrome. An example is over-excitement with fluoxetine treatment in a child with autism.

4. **Due to other factors:** The behaviour may be unrelated to the syndrome directly. An example would be disturbed behaviour reflecting family trauma of a child with autism. The child's condition, however, may make them more susceptible to external influences.

In this chapter we discuss five categories of syndrome: Genetic, Epileptic, Developmental, Teratogenic, and Mental Health. The distinction between these is somewhat arbitrary and the syndromes described are illustrative rather than comprehensive.

Genetic syndromes

Consider a child with Prader–Willi syndrome (PWS). Specific to that condition are a set of behaviours not otherwise explained by general developmental and environmental understandings. Such behaviours include severe hyperphagia, 'obsessive' behaviours, and risk of rage-like tantrums.

Behaviours more likely in individuals with a particular genetic disorder are termed 'behavioural phenotypes'. These features can be included as Predisposing factors in the 5P model. There may be syndrome-specific treatment strategies (e.g. for PWS (1)).

With whole-exome and whole-genome genetic profiling available, many genetic anomalies are being identified. In many cases these are assumed to be causal, in others the significance of the finding is less certain. Even for causal genetic findings, the genotype–phenotype relationship may remain uncertain. This is usually because too few cases have been described to allow valid definition of behavioural phenotype.

Although a genetic syndrome diagnosis may not change management of behaviour, there may still be value in pursuing aetiological diagnosis with genetic testing—in providing family support, clearing up misunderstandings, alleviating guilt, and providing families access to emerging new treatments. Also, establishing a genetic diagnosis helps to build knowledge and information about behavioural phenotypes.

We have summarized some of the common syndromes and their behavioural phenotypes in Appendix 6.1. For further information on these, and other syndromes, see the syndrome fact sheets provided by the Society for the Study of Behavioural Phenotypes (SSBP).[1]

Epilepsy

Epilepsy, defined as two or more unprovoked seizures, occurs more commonly in children with developmental disabilities.

It is generally possible to gather clinical data to help determine if seizures (e.g. complex partial) may be responsible for particular behaviour. Differences between seizure and non-seizure behaviours are summarized in Table 6.1.

Differentiating seizure-related behaviour from other causes can be challenging. A 2010 study in the United Kingdom (2) found that around one-third of individuals with ID, later shown to have epilepsy, had previous misdiagnoses. These misdiagnoses were a consequence of the misinterpretation of behavioural, physiological, syndrome-related, medication-related, or psychological events by parents, paid carers, and health professionals.

Another behavioural pattern seen in this population is that of increasing irritability and aggression often over a period of 2 to 3 weeks, culminating in a

---

[1] Society for the Study of Behavioural Phenotypes. https://ssbp.org.uk/syndrome-she ets/. Accessed September 30 2025.

Table 6.1 Epileptic compared to non-epileptic aggressive behaviour

Epileptic	Non-epileptic
Child is confused or disoriented	Child appears normally alert and oriented
Aggression is disorganized (e.g. flailing arms)	Aggression is organized, planned, more complex, more purposeful
Generally, no trigger	Often occurs in well-known context (e.g. denial of wanted activity or object)
May be preceded by changed non-aggressive mental state	Sometimes preceded by progressive increase in agitation
Often sudden onset	May be gradual onset
May end in sleep	Usually doesn't end with sleep
Sequence and time course of behaviour disturbance tends to be stereotyped	Often more variable in pattern and time course

grand mal fit. Following the seizure, irritability declines. After a variable time period the cycle is repeated. This can prove challenging to treat. Antipsychotics may reduce the irritability but lower seizure threshold. Anticonvulsants may have the opposite effects.

If this escalation/resolution pattern is suspected, a daily diary is useful, recording irritability symptoms, episodes of convulsions, and effects of medication changes. The resulting chart will demonstrate whether the temporal relationship of aggression and convulsions conforms to the cyclical syndrome. Electroencephalogram (EEG) telemetry over time may help with correlation of behaviour and electrical activity.

In addition to seizures impacting behaviour, anticonvulsant medication may be causal. Benzodiazepines frequently cause disinhibition or irritability. Anti-epileptic medications more generally may cause agitation, aggression, psychosis, disruptive behaviour, hyperactivity, and restlessness. Anti-epileptic medication may also improve behaviour, particularly in situations where behaviour is associated with dysregulated mood.

Psychogenic, non-epileptic seizures are discussed under Somatic and Conversion disorders.

Developmental syndromes

Under this heading, we group a set of disorders with the following in common:

1. They are diagnosed on clinical criteria.

2. The disorders are generally dimensional, such that diagnostic boundaries are based on clinical judgement and statistical properties of assessment tools.

3. Behaviours that comprised the diagnostic criteria may be considered normal at a younger age but persist beyond age norms.

4. Within a diagnosed group of children there is likely to be substantial heterogeneity in both clinical phenotype and severity.

5. The biological basis of the disorder may not be clearly established.

When the biological cause of the developmental disorder is not well defined, several consequences may arise:

- Different people involved in the child's care may have different explanations of a child's behaviour, for example that the child is not trying hard enough, or has a bad attitude, or that the behaviour is chosen by the child to be disruptive.

- There may be unrealistic expectations about treatment outcomes in the short term (neuroplasticity) and longer term (natural history).

Across all developmental syndromes, children struggle with resulting impairments, such as difficulties in learning and communication. In addition, children may suffer from the consequences of how their problems are understood and managed. Clarity around the biological underpinnings of the child's disorder, even when this is not fully established, can serve to reduce this second area of potential harm, enabling understanding and expectation that is closer to the truth for the child.

Attention Deficit Hyperactivity Disorder

Practice guidelines regarding Attention Deficit Hyperactivity Disorder (ADHD) have been developed in a number of countries (see Table 6.2). All these indicate that pharmacological treatment of ADHD has been shown to be effective in the short term for the core symptoms of ADHD, particularly disordered attention control, impulsivity, and hyperactivity. Paediatricians may consult these.

When using medication, consider the following with regards to problematic behaviour:

- Medication may be effective, but only partially.

- Time-related variability, for example when the medication wears off.

- Medication side effects, for example depressed mood, emotional volatility.

Table 6.2 National and international consensus guidelines for ADHD

International	The World Federation of ADHD International Consensus Statement: 208 Evidence-based conclusions about the disorder. https://doi.org/10.1016/j.neubiorev.2021.01.022. Published September 2021. Accessed Sept 30 2025.
USA	American Academy of Pediatrics, Subcommittee on Children and Adolescents with Attention-Deficit/Hyperactivity Disorder. ADHD: Clinical practice guideline for the diagnosis, evaluation, and treatment of children and adolescents with attention-deficit/hyperactivity disorder. Pediatrics, 30 September 2019. Society for Developmental and Behavioral Pediatrics clinical practice guideline for the assessment and treatment of children and adolescents with complex attention-deficit/hyperactivity disorder. J Dev Behav Pediatr. 2020 Feb-Mar; 41: S35–S57. | DOI: 10.1097/DBP.0000000000000770. https://journals.lww.com/jrnldbp/fulltext/2020/03001/society_for_developmental_and_behavioral.3.aspx.
Canada	Canadian ADHD Practice Guidelines 4.1. Published January 2020. Accessed Sept 30 2025. https://www.caddra.ca/canadian-adhd-practice-guidelines/.
UK	NICE Guidelines: Attention Deficit Hyperactivity Disorder: Diagnosis and Management. https://www.nice.org.uk/guidance/ng87/resources/attention-deficit-hyperactivity-disorder-diagnosis-and-management-pdf-1837699732933. Published March 2018. Accessed Sept 30 2025.
Australia	Australian Evidence-Based Clinical Practice Guideline for Attention Deficit Hyperactivity Disorder (ADHD) 1st edition. https://adhdguideline.aadpa.com.au/download/. Published October 2022. Accessed Sept 30 2025.

In addition, consider:

- Comorbid problems, for example problems of emotional control;

- How the problem is managed, for example frustration arising due to expectations of the child they are unable to meet; and

- The life experience of the child, for example bullying.

Medication may make it easier for children to think before acting, but it does not direct the choices they make. Rather than considering medication as 'treating the behaviour', ADHD medications can be seen as medical modification of neurological control systems (e.g. impulse control). Further intervention may be required to help the child learn more adaptive behaviours in the opportunity created through better control. This approach of using medication to 'enable' as well as 'treat' is particularly useful in ADHD.

ADHD and emotional control

ADHD often co-occurs with disordered emotional control (anxiety, irritability, depressed mood, and Obsessive-Compulsive Disorder (OCD)). For some children, ADHD may seem 'primary' and the associated behaviours 'secondary'. Treating the ADHD successfully may lead to gratifying resolution of the associated behaviours.

For many others, ADHD treatment may be of limited benefit in altering behaviour problems, or may cause side effects. For these children, successful treatment outcomes may necessitate stabilizing emotional control and treating the co-occurring condition first. Clinical judgement is likely to guide how best to sequence the treatment approach for these children.

Anxiety

ADHD is a stressful condition that may provoke secondary anxiety. To reduce anxiety, initial management should include explanation. A trial of stimulant medication is reasonable, as it may help the child experience a more predictable life. If the anxiety resolves, this supports the hypothesis that anxiety is secondary. If trials of stimulants are not helpful, atomoxetine may be useful. Persistent and impairing anxiety warrants cognitive behavioural therapy (CBT) as noted in Chapter 5, and further consideration of evidence-based pharmacotherapy with SSRI medication.

Depression

Persistent irritability and depressed mood in children with ADHD may indicate comorbid depression. Where the cause is not clear, and the depression is embedded, an opinion from a psychiatrist is suggested. Depression and impulse control problems add independent risk of self-harm. Where appropriate, consider pharmacotherapy for depression if symptoms are severe or if there is inadequate response to psychotherapy. ADHD medications are more likely to be helpful in addressing ADHD-related behaviours once the depression has improved.

Mood instability

Mood instability in children with ADHD may reflect impulsive, reactive, and oppositional outbursts. They may also be a manifestation of depression or Disruptive Mood Dysregulation Disorder, or a response to environmental stressors. Thorough assessment as outlined in Chapter 4 is essential to guide holistic management. A trial of stimulant medication may lead to prompt resolution of mood instability. Conversely, it may increase irritability. Monitoring the behaviours over time and in response to treatment may give the paediatrician additional insights and strengthen the diagnostic formulation.

Tics and OCD

Tic disorders and OCD occur commonly in children with ADHD, and 50% of all children with tic disorders have ADHD (3). Stimulants are not contraindicated in children with tic disorders. Response is variable, including worsening or improvement in tics. A guiding principle for the clinician is to prioritize treatment goals with the child and family through a process of shared decision-making. If treating tics is a priority, it may be advisable to use clonidine or guanfacine as a first-line medication and consider referral for Comprehensive Behavioural Intervention for Tics (CBIT)/habit reversal.

ADHD with Intellectual Disability

For children with ID, there is a danger of overdiagnosis of ADHD. DSM-5 and ICD-11 require that symptoms of ADHD are necessarily judged against the child's developmental age, rather than chronological age. Even when the diagnosis is appropriate, the benefits of stimulant medications may be more modest than expected.

ADHD and social development

ADHD may be associated with impairments of social understanding in two ways. For social learning, children need to pay attention to salient social information, to store the learnings from social interactions, and to retrieve and utilize these learnings in new situations. The executive function impairments associated with ADHD may hinder this developmental learning on a cumulative basis over time. As a result, social learning lags increasingly behind age expectations, an acquired developmental delay. A second association occurs because comorbidity of Autism Spectrum Disorder (ASD) with ADHD occurs at greater frequency than background risk for either condition (4).

In both cases (delay and/or disorder), medical treatment of ADHD may lead to better self-control (e.g. capacity to think before acting) but is unlikely to substantially alter behaviours that arise from the social impairments directly. Instead, we recommend using medical treatment to enable more successful interventions for those children whose capacity to learn is hindered by problems of impulse and attention control. Whilst doing this, it is important to ensure that behavioural strategy is adjusted to the child's 'social developmental age' rather than default for chronological age.

> ## Practice tip. ADHD and behaviour problems
>
> Given the frequency and range of developmental issues comorbid with ADHD, management of associated behaviour problems will be more successful if undertaken with a comprehensive formulation to identify the full set of potential contributing factors.

Pharmacological treatment of ADHD

Although guidelines recommend standard dosing protocols, we have observed substantial variability in child response when ADHD is associated with other disorders (5). This may reflect differences in brain function.

For this reason, a 'low and slow' approach is recommended, beginning with the smallest amount regardless of age (e.g. half a tablet), grading up slowly (interval depending on medication half-life). Such an approach is particularly important for medications with longer half-lives, such as atomoxetine, as it is otherwise easy to 'overshoot' the optimal dosage.

As noted above, successful medical treatment also creates greater opportunity for learning for those children whose capacity to learn is hindered by poor attention and impulse control. Choice of medication, dose, and timing should consider optimizing opportunities for remediation as well as behavioural support. When remediation has been achieved, the use of medication should be reviewed.

Autism

We assume paediatricians are already familiar with the diagnosis and management of autism. Consensus guidelines are listed below (Table 6.3). Here we discuss areas of behaviour associated with this diagnosis that are likely to be a clinical challenge for paediatricians.

A diagnosis of autism or ASD may provide potential access to support interventions. In the United Kingdom, there was an almost eightfold increase in diagnosis rates for ASD in the 20 years from 1998 to 2018 (6). Prevalence amongst children in the United States has risen to around 3% (7). Similar increases are reported in Canada and Australia. Debate continues whether this represents increased detection of genuine, mostly milder ASD, or over-diagnosis for reasons such as funding incentives and algorithmic diagnostic methodologies (8).

Table 6.3 National consensus guidelines for ASD

UK	National Institute for Health and Care Excellence. Autism spectrum disorder in under 19s: Recognition, referral and diagnosis. Clinical guideline [CG128] Last updated: 20 December 2017. CG128 was Published September 2011, accessed 10/04/2025, https://www.nice.org.uk/guidance/cg128 National Institute for Health and Care Excellence. Autism spectrum disorder in under 19s: support and management. Clinical guideline [CG170] Last updated: 14 June 2021. CG170 was Published August 2013, accessed 10/04/2025, https://www.nice.org.uk/guidance/cg170
USA	American Academy of Pediatrics. Hyman SL et al. Identification, evaluation, and management of children with autism spectrum disorder. Pediatrics 2020;145(1):e20193447. https://doi.org/10.1542/peds.2019-3447.
Canada	Canadian Paediatric Society: Standards of diagnostic assessment for autism spectrum disorder (October 2019). Early detection for autism spectrum disorder in young children (October 2019). Post-diagnostic management and follow-up care for autism spectrum disorder (October 2019).
Australia	Autism CRC: Whitehouse AJO, Evans K, Eapen V, Wray J. A national guideline for the assessment and diagnosis of autism spectrum disorders in Australia. Cooperative Research Centre for Living with Autism, Brisbane, 2018. Autism CRC: Trembath, D et al. National guideline for supporting the learning, participation, and wellbeing of autistic children and their families in Australia. Cooperative Research Centre for Living with Autism, Brisbane, 2022.

When children have complex behavioural problems such as those encountered in autism, and particularly when a diagnosis enables access to intervention supports, there may be a tension between diagnostic reductionism and a full bio-psycho-social formulation of the child's predicament. This challenge of diagnosis in situations of clinical complexity and uncertainty is one confronting every paediatrician (9). A risk is that all behaviour problems may be attributed to the ASD diagnosis, rather than additional comorbid factors such as trauma. Intervention strategy may default to pre-specified ASD algorithmic treatments. The paediatrician has an important role in keeping a child's individual set of problems in the foreground.

Behavioural interventions

Use of standardized behaviourally based skill development interventions is common for ASD. Examples include Applied Behaviour Analysis (ABA) and the Early Start Denver Model (ESDM). The Paediatrician still has an important role:

- **Overview of priorities**: Priorities reflect what is important for the child and family. This includes the amount of therapy (sustainable workload) as well as the intended purposes of intervention.

- **Overview of progress**: Progress is built around setting expected treatment outcome goals, then reviewing them. If goals have not been achieved, the underlying assumptions should be reviewed.

- **Medical advocacy**: Not all problems are readily amenable to behavioural interventions. The child who is highly and recurrently distressed, for example, may even be harmed by behavioural strategies.

- **Strengths and interests**: Behavioural interventions run the risk of being both standardized in nature and deficit-remedial in purpose. This minimizes the extent to which the child's voice is heard. What is the child's purpose? What interests and motivates them?

Clinical heterogeneity

The diagnostic systems DSM-5 and ICD-11 consider behaviours in social-communicative and restricted interests groupings. A diagnostic category implies a degree of diagnostic homogeneity. However, children who meet diagnostic criteria for ASD diagnosis are heterogeneous, particularly regarding associated behaviour.

- **Biological and clinical variability**: Each child has a different combination of intensity of impairment in language, sociability, sensory disturbance, restricted interests, and repetitive behaviours. Further, the full range of intellectual function can be seen, from superior intelligence to profound intellectual disability. Some children have savant skills, though these often do not contribute strongly to adaptive function.

- **Psychosocial variability**: Each child with autism develops in the context of a unique family, with a unique experience that may range from loving and nurturing to rejection and abuse. The school experience also varies greatly. Some children are educated in specialized autism settings which are highly attuned to their needs, while others are unable to find a suitable educational arrangement.

For these reasons we recommend that clinical care, including management of difficult behaviour, be individualized according to the guiding principles we have discussed. Standardized therapeutic techniques are generally derived from group-level research. The children in this research may be atypically homogeneous because of enrolment exclusions. In clinical practice, a bespoke formulation is needed to determine optimal treatment for each child.

Practice tip: Behavioural formulation when a child has ASD

Diagnosis of ASD is insufficient by itself to guide an appropriate management plan. What is needed is comprehensive formulation of the child's:

- Autism symptoms (individual for that child)

- Intellectual and cognitive profile

- Communication skills

- Self-control capacity (attention, impulse, emotional)

- Behaviours

- Interests and strengths

- Family function

- School function

'High-functioning' autism in the school years

Intelligent children with autism frequently do not fit easily into autism-specific classes when other children in the class have various levels of intellectual disability. For this reason, attempts are frequently made to enrol them in mainstream regular classes. In these settings, however, the children may struggle because:

- Their level of social comprehension and related behavioural function may be expected to be similar to their intellectual level, when it is not.

- Idiosyncrasies of interest and behaviour are obvious to the typically developing children, and this makes the child the frequent target of teasing and bullying.

- The sensory environment, particularly events with large numbers of children (e.g. sporting events, assembly), may be overwhelming.

The consequences may be substantial distress to the autistic child. In the absence of capacity to find better educational fit, home schooling may substantially improve the well-being of such a child.

Practice tip: Bullying

Teasing or bullying of children with autism in regular school settings is so common that it can be used as a screening question. Other children see those with autism as 'weird' and inevitably let them know.

An important function of the paediatrician is to encourage parents to be vigilant in protecting their autistic child from bullying, and to assist them in advocacy with school for this purpose.

Everyday life stressors

Life for a child with ASD may be recurrently distressing. The child may struggle to understand social situations and messages, perceiving situations of uncertainty as threat. They may find the sensory load of situations overwhelming, particularly sound. Even in situations they understand and can manage, their biological control of emotional responses may produce responses to everyday situations that are disproportionate.

In addition to the impact these responses have on quality of life, stressors may serve to interfere with the child's participation in life, and capacity for learning. They are often the driving energy behind difficult behaviour. In situations where everyday life stressors drive difficult behaviour, management follows the presumed causal hypothesis:

1. As much as possible, reduce the uncertainty in a child's life. This may include avoidance of potentially problematic situations, or strategies to prepare the child for what is coming.

2. As much as possible, consider the child's sensory experience, keeping this compatible with sensory preferences, predictable and stable.

3. Consider the total 'workload' for the child. A reduced set of activities may enable the child to sustainably manage without undue fatigue.

4. At a behavioural level, try to build capacity to manage difficult situations, for example through repeated graded exposure.

5. Where emotional responses are still the driving force for harmful consequences, consider the use of psychotropic medication.

Over-arousal, agitation, irritability

Children with ASD may have agitation that presents similarly to ADHD symptoms. When the drivers for activation behaviours cannot be identified or altered
at an environmental level, medication may be a useful adjunct to modifying
these. The goal is for children to be sufficiently settled that they gain the most
benefit from associated therapeutic and support strategies.

Major tranquilizers such as risperidone, olanzapine, and quetiapine are useful
for this set of activation symptoms. These all have the side effects of weight
gain and hyperprolactinemia to a variable degree. Aripiprazole and lurasidone
sometimes produce less of these side effects. In some countries, access to the
newer antipsychotic medications may be difficult. The older combination of
haloperidol combined if necessary, with benztropine may have a role as it
causes little weight gain and is inexpensive.

The alpha-adrenergic drugs clonidine and guanfacine can also modify over-
arousal. However, their effects may wear off after a few weeks or months. This
may be restored with a break of a week or so. They require reliable caregivers
because sudden cessation can cause rebound hypertension, and overdosage of
these medications may be harmful to the child.

Repetitive behaviours: Obsessions, preoccupations, rituals, stereotypical movements

The first step is to assess the impact of these behaviours on the child's well-
being. If the behaviours are not causing significant impairment, it is reasonable
to tolerate or redirect them.

Restrictive and repetitive behaviours (RRBs) are usually resistant to reward
strategies. When rituals or preoccupations are problematic, Selective Serotonin
Reuptake Inhibitors (SSRI) medications are often considered. Research regarding their use has two important findings.

1. SSRI medications have generally been disappointing in achieving reduction
   in the frequency of spontaneous RRBs (10).

2. At the same time, parents often report that children are more easily diverted
   from RRBs. It is presumed this is a consequence of reduced anxiety. In our
   experience, SSRIs can be beneficial when used in this way.

A group of repetitive movements, sometimes called 'stimming' can be managed with the same considerations. As noted above, SSRIs may enable greater
capacity for behavioural diversion.

What are termed 'obsessions' in autism are more accurately described as 'preoccupations'. As explained below in the discussion of Obsessive-Compulsive Disorder, autistic preoccupations do not have the properties of true obsessions.

Restricted diet, avoidant/restrictive food intake disorder (ARFID)

Food-related behaviours, restrictive in range or quantity are common amongst children diagnosed with ASD. More extreme behaviours may lead to problems of nutrition and growth. Management depends on the nature of the food restriction. Examples include:

- Texture—change when possible (e.g. from solids to semi-solid).

- Taste and smell—find dietary alternatives.

- Volume—very small amounts, repeated.

- Aversion due to previous experience—change how food is presented (e.g. blended with foods the child likes).

- Control—do not make food a battle. Dinner is a time for social connectedness as well as eating.

- Hunger—if a child snacks when hungry, they are unlikely to have substantial appetite for meals.

- Encouragement—eating behaviours can be incentivized by rewards (e.g. desired foods, activities) following small achievable acts of eating bravery. This is more likely to be successful if the child is involved in choosing both the incentivized behaviour (e.g. a single vegetable) and associated rewards.

Paediatricians will detect if a child is nutritionally compromised and provide reassurance when they are not. As with Anorexia Nervosa, more extreme cases are likely to need specialized expertise. A benefit of some psychotropic medications (e.g. mirtazapine, antipsychotics) may be increased appetite.

Use of medication in ASD

In situations where the clinical symptoms interfere with function and quality of life, and have proven resistant to non-pharmacological treatments, the following medications may be useful. If medication is used as an adjunct and enabler for behavioural therapy, it is important to clarify purpose and associated expectations. As with the discussion around repetitive behaviours above, medication may not substantially alter behaviour directly. Instead, medication for anxious children may modify the 'malleability' of a situation, enabling more successful non-medical therapy.

Table 6.4 Summary of medications used in ASD

Clinical challenge	Psychotropic medications to consider
Problematic hyperactivity, inattention, distractibility	ADHD medications—e.g. stimulants
Persisting problems of sleep onset	Melatonin
Problematic inflexibility in rituals, obsessions	SSRIs
Significant dysfunction due to sensory sensitivities	Atypical antipsychotics—mainly prn usage
Overarousal, agitation	Atypical antipsychotics Alpha-adrenergic agonists, e.g. clonidine
Dysphoria, depression	SSRIs, mirtazapine

Intermittent (prn) medication

Day-to-day behaviour problems in autism can often be minimized using sedatives or tranquilizers on a prn basis. The advantage of this approach is that side effects are generally much less when medications are used episodically rather than on a continuous daily basis. The paediatrician and the family can trial either a sedative such as diazepam or an antipsychotic such as risperidone in different doses to determine the best effect.

This approach is most useful when families know and can predict situations which reliably cause major distress for their child with autism and are not amenable to a contextual or behavioural intervention. In that case, the medication can be given as a one-off 30 minutes before the situation arises. Examples might be a child who becomes very distressed:

- when they have to have their hair or nails cut

- when they have to travel on a plane

- when a visit to a noisy or crowded place is unavoidable

Many families have reported that this approach has made the family's life much more tolerable and less stressful.

Intellectual Disability

The relationship of Intellectual Disability (ID) to associated behaviour needs to be understood in terms of each child's developmental age. If a 10-year-old child functions at a 3-year-old level, understanding and management of that child's behaviour should also be modified to a 3-year-old level.

Behaviour problems are 2 to 3 times more common in children with ID than in typically developing children. Around 40% of children and adolescents with ID have major behaviour problems. This excess of behaviour problems appears in infancy and continues through life (11). The severity of behaviour problems appears to decline gradually after about the third decade. The impact of the behaviour problems on those around the child with ID increases through adolescence as the child gets bigger.

Practice tip: Intellectual disability does not cause behaviour problems

All behaviour problems in children with ID are caused by factors other than the ID itself (with the exception of the situation described below). It is the task of assessment and formulation to discover these other factors.

The only situation in which behaviour problems can be directly attributable to ID is where a child has behaviour which is normal for a child of his mental age, but because of being physically older and larger, the behaviour causes problems for others. For example, a boy of 16 who has severe ID may have tantrums which are typical of a child of his mental age of 3 years. However, these tantrums are a problem because his physical size means injury or damage can occur during the tantrum.

The term 'diagnostic overshadowing' was first introduced to describe the tendency to falsely attribute all behaviour problems in a child with ID to the ID itself, ignoring the real causative factors.

Why are behaviour problems so common in children with ID? There are three principal reasons:

1. Healthy behaviour requires a healthy brain. In ID, the brain is not working normally in various ways beyond the impact on cognition.

2. Intelligence conveys a capacity to find adaptive solutions to life challenges. This capacity is not available to individuals with ID to the same extent as typically developing children.

3. Children with ID suffer increased rates of deprivation and abuse of all types. Families of children with ID experience poverty to an increased degree.

Poverty itself increases rates of behaviour problems, largely through living in adverse neighbourhoods.

Behaviour problems vary in type according to the severity of ID. Those with mild ID have psychopathology similar to non-ID children, although with cognitively simpler content. Those with moderate and severe ID display behaviours which are rarely seen in non-ID children, such as rocking or head banging and the autistic symptoms. Children with profound ID have fewer behaviour problems, largely because they have a limited repertoire of behaviour (see Rutter's Child and Adolescent Psychiatry, pp. 820–840 (12).

As discussed in Chapter 3, there are specific instruments which have been developed to assess behaviour problems in children with intellectual disability. These include the Developmental Behaviour Checklist and the Aberrant Behaviour Checklist.

Even with reasonable support, the individual may not understand communications or expectations. Problem behaviour may indicate that the child is distressed, confused, or feels unsafe and frightened. They may just be upset because they cannot have what they want or successfully communicate their needs. For that reason, it is important for the paediatrician to understand the situation from the child's perspective, as well as working to manage the behaviour itself.

The interaction of ID and specific mental health problems is discussed later in this chapter.

Borderline intellectual function

The plight of children with borderline ID (e.g. IQ 70–80) is worthy of specific mention. This group is at increased risk for mental health and behavioural problems compared with the average child (13). Borderline intellectual function places children in a difficult situation. They are not formally identified as intellectually disabled and may not meet criteria for formally funded and structured support. Capacity to learn, however, is likely to fall below the level expected in life generally, academic curriculum and social context specifically. This challenge is likely to increase as curriculum and life generally becomes more complex and abstract.

With academic curriculum and life more generally, expectations need to be adapted as appropriate. It is unfair and unreasonable to expect these children to manage an unmodified curriculum.

Health issues

Medical care of behaviour for individuals with ID includes addressing factors such as sleep disturbances, seizures, and gut dysfunction, especially constipation. When behaviour problems appear *de novo* in a non-verbal child, it is particularly important to search for sources of pain. The most common hidden sources are dental problems and abdominal pain (see Chapter 2).

Social context

There is a strong association between mild ID and socio-economic disadvantage, because mild ID has a strong genetic component. As an independent risk factor, economic and social disadvantage substantially increases the rate of behaviour problems (14). This is associated with neighbourhood experience (e.g. crime, violence, drug abuse), behavioural modelling, and threat associated with uncertainty. Children with ID have less intellectual capacity to manage these challenges.

Specific Learning Disorders

Specific Learning Disorders (SLD) are common, and it is expected the paediatrician will have a working understanding in the detection, diagnosis and management of these (15). As with ID, there are no behaviour problems intrinsic to SLD. The increased likelihood of problem behaviour arises from how the child adapts to having an SLD.

From the child's point of view, having an SLD that is not well managed generates stress from the mismatch between expectations and the child's capacity. Behaviour problems arise from the child's response to this predicament. Temperamentally sensitive children may become more anxious, avoidant, or withdrawn. Agitated children may become oppositional or aggressive. Impulsive children may become the 'class clown', acting up for attention or the perceived admiration of their peers.

When children present with behaviour problems of uncertain causation, we recommend consideration of underlying SLD that may not have been formally identified. This is particularly so for those in secondary education.

Management of maladaptive behaviours is unlikely to be successful without first correcting the goodness of fit between capacity and expectations. Children with SLD need to feel safe and able to achieve predictably and sustainably what is expected of them. Only then is it appropriate to consider supports (e.g. tutoring) intended to build learning capacity, and interventions to modify the adaptive behaviours.

SLD has a strong comorbidity with ADHD (16). The clinical impact of ADHD often extends to learning (17). SLD may occur within a diagnosed condition with more widespread impact (e.g. consequences of FASD, mathematics in Turner syndrome, reading comprehension in some children with ASD). The learning consequences of possible SLD in these situations are an important consideration when understanding and managing behaviour problems.

Motor control disorders

As with ID and SLD, problems of motor control and function do not cause problem behaviour. The relation between motor problems and behaviour may be due to:

- Fatigue, particularly when behaviour problems increase during the waking hours.

- Anxiety and desire for avoidance, particularly if children have been shamed and teased for their impaired motor capacities. This may be particularly so for team sports and other physical activities where poor coordination and skills are evident to peers.

Whether Developmental Coordination Disorder (DCD) or Cerebral Palsy (CP), the challenge for children is fundamentally the same. Movement (and associated functional skills) is more difficult to plan, undertake, habituate, and sustain than would otherwise be expected for intellectual and general developmental level.

As with other developmental challenges, managing behaviour may be unsuccessful until the underlying predicament for the child is appropriately addressed. Good medical care may include finding what the child might be able to do (e.g. individual or cooperative activities rather than team sports) and working towards competencies that enable meaningful physical participation. Maintaining movement and physical health generally makes a positive difference with all developmental problems and associated behaviours.

Tic disorders

Tics are common in children with developmental disorders. By definition, tics are not premeditated, so standard behavioural strategy is inappropriate.

Whilst tics are unusual, they are not generally behaviours that cause direct harm for children, beyond embarrassment and social consequences. If tics themselves are problematic for children at a behavioural level, tic-specific behavioural interventions that combine elements of habit reversal training with psychoeducation may be useful, for example CBIT and Habit Reversal Therapy (HRT) (18). Management includes consideration of situational risk (when the child is tired, stressed, or relaxing). Beyond these strategies, medication to reduce tic intensity may be a reasonable consideration. Recent clinical guidelines outline a step-by-step approach to tic management (19).

Beyond tics, the 'Tourette Syndrome cluster' is commonly associated with problems of executive function/ADHD, and anxiety/OCD (20). Management of these associated problems may be of equal if not greater benefit to the child generally, and specifically towards reduction in problematic behaviour.

Stereotypic movements

Stereotypic movement behaviours are repetitive and seemingly purposeless. Examples include shaking, hand-waving or flapping, rocking, and hitting oneself. They occur more frequently in individuals who have more severe biologically based problems, such as ASD and moderate to profound ID, and often manifest early in development.

Some parents are embarrassed by their child's stereotypic movements in public environments as they are an easily observed sign of behavioural anomaly.

Behaviours leading to direct harm are referred to as Self-Injurious Behaviours (SIB). Beyond the direct harm, SIB can be particularly distressing for parents and caregivers, particularly due to their resistance to treatment. Harm minimization with helmets, gloves, and other physical blockage strategies are often necessary.

From a behaviour perspective, the management goal is to reduce direct (e.g. self-hitting) and indirect harm (e.g. impairments of function and development). Like any other behaviour problem, management commences with a comprehensive assessment. Particularly pertinent is 'analysis of contextual variation', discussed in Chapter 3, as these behaviours nearly always vary in intensity or occurrence in time or context. This will frequently give a clue to exacerbating or ameliorating strategies. For example, there may be agreement between observers that the stereotypic behaviour occurs when the child appears to be bored. This can then be tested by replacing a bored period with one with increased stimulation and measuring whether the frequency of the stereotypy declines.

Where contextual variation is unclear, or as an adjunct to modifying environment (context), a common behavioural strategy used is Differential Reinforcement of Other Behaviours (DRO). This is a positive reinforcement method that rewards more adaptive behaviours.

Another behavioural approach for children with greater capacity for self-awareness and communication is Functional Communication Training (FTC), which teaches and rewards communication strategy that enables the child to replace stereotypical movements with other communication methods when they are aware that they need something or are feeling distressed.

Other movements which may resemble stereotypies are

- Tics

- Extrapyramidal syndromes, often drug-induced

◆ Catatonia

◆ Seizures

Sometimes the distinction between these movements may be difficult. Tics are generally sudden, discontinuous, nonrhythmic, and may commence later in life. Consultation with a neurologist may be indicated to differentiate these presentations.

Medication treatments for self-injurious behaviour tend to be empirical. One tries different psychotropics in the hope that something helps. Antipsychotics are the most often useful. Clonidine may help. Naltrexone has been tried but rarely works in our experience. Benzodiazepines may be useful, especially lorazepam in catatonia.

Sleep–wake disorders

Disturbances of sleep and circadian control are recognized as a group of problems in DSM-5. They are more common in children who have developmental disorders than the general population. Whilst sleep disturbance may not be considered a behavioural problem, it has considerable negative impact on those who care for the child, as well as the child themselves. This may be due to fatigue as well as associated behaviours (e.g. desire for Internet game play during the night).

As with motor problems, sleep-related problems may be overlooked in children who have significant developmental and behavioural disorders. Milder problems may be managed with good sleep hygiene. It is our expectation that each paediatrician will have medications they use to modify sleep-related function (e.g. clonidine). There is evidence from systematic reviews that melatonin is safe and efficacious in children with developmental disabilities (21, 22). Its main effect is to reduce sleep-onset latency.

Orexin agonists (suvorexant, lemborexant) are newer hypnotics. At the time of writing, literature on their use in children with developmental disabilities is limited to open-label case studies.

Where medication is used, we recommend this be combined with behaviourally based sleep strategy towards the goal of medication minimization and eventual cessation if possible.

A sleep diary (onset, morning waking, additional sleep/waking episodes) is likely to be of benefit, particularly for viewing patterns that occur over several days or weeks. Sleep studies may otherwise be necessary for problems associated with seizures, airways obstruction, and respiratory problems.

From the mildest annoying behaviours associated with ADHD, through to the most distressing and disruptive behaviours in children with ASD and ID, correcting disturbances of sleep as much as possible can sometimes be an easy 'win', an intervention with quick and potentially substantial benefit.

Teratogenic syndromes

Teratogenic syndromes result from damage to a previously healthy biology, particularly the central nervous system. Examples include infections, brain injury, and damage from toxins such as intrauterine alcohol exposure.

In general, damage is a time-limited event, with subsequent continuing consequences. Where damage is ongoing (e.g. neurodegenerative disorders), the developmental and behavioural consequences change correspondingly over time. Beyond the medical management of neurological pathology, it is of particular importance to consider the child's experience, function, quality of life, and learning, even when these are changing over time.

Some teratogenic processes have predictable consequences. Examples include the risk of sensory deficits in congenital rubella, or global reduction in cognitive capacity in cases of lead toxicity. Otherwise, the impact of teratogens is variable, for example the child with brain injury from trauma or infection. Management then requires understanding of children on an individual basis. This may be achieved with comprehensive neuropsychological assessment, interpreted in terms of the competencies necessary for comprehension, behavioural control, and learning. To consider behaviour in the context of teratogenic damage, we discuss the example of intrauterine alcohol.

Foetal Alcohol Spectrum Disorder

In Australia, Foetal Alcohol Spectrum Disorder (FASD) is the most common preventable cause of brain injury in children (23). It is a serious problem not only for children and families but also the community as a whole. Whilst we discuss management of attributable behaviours, we acknowledge the profound importance of public health measures directed towards prevention, harm reduction, early detection, and intervention.

The challenge for children diagnosed with FASD is likely to be multifactorial due to the increased likelihood of additional toxicity (substance use during pregnancy) along with the impact of adverse perinatal/postnatal experiences which are more likely in this group (24).

FASD leads to lifelong developmental, behavioural, and mental health consequences. The pattern of injury, and consequences for both function and behaviour, relate both to the distribution and timing of damage. However, it is generally difficult to predict the extent, and pattern of consequences, from the alcohol ingestion history. The history of antenatal alcohol use is often unattainable or unreliable. As an intrauterine process of damage, FASD potentially affects not only all aspects of the central nervous system but all organs of the body (25).

When FASD is associated with behaviour problems, the clinical challenge is to understand how all associated impairments relate to the child's behaviour. Consideration includes the child's general cognition, specific learning, social comprehension, emotional regulation (anxiety, temper, threat responses), capacity to communicate, and particularly self-control (executive function). Such an understanding informs what is likely to be possible with standard behaviour management strategy, and how to deal with situations where this is not the case.

A common behavioural challenge identified for children with FASD is that they do not seem to 'learn from their mistakes'. Problem behaviour persists despite management that is seeming appropriate. In this situation there is a risk of attributing this persistence to wilful misbehaviour. Instead, it is more likely due to combined impairments, particularly those of executive function and learning (26). The result of this is that a child has difficulty both learning and retaining what is expected, retrieving that information in situations where it is necessary, and maintaining the self-control to put this information into behavioural choice. Appropriate management addresses both issues, the child's capacity to understand and learn as well as capacity to retrieve and use this information in appropriate situations. The paediatrician's role in this includes medication, parental education and support, and advocacy (e.g. with education staff).

There is no 'medication for FASD'. Choice of medication is guided by clinical information, and the overall formulation to explain behaviour. Common targets for medication are impulsivity, executive function more generally, anxiety, and other disorders of mood regulation.

Mental health syndromes

Mental disorders occur more commonly in children who have developmental disability than in the general population (27). We address this in some detail as paediatricians report this area of clinical practice as a gap in their training. In this book we use the terms 'psychiatric', 'mental health', and 'mental disorder' somewhat interchangeably.

Symptoms, syndromes, and mental disorders

The terminology of challenging behaviour can be confusing, particularly the relationship between 'behaviour problems' and 'psychiatric problems'. There is no valid distinction between these as categories. In this book, we regard behaviours viewed at the symptom level as equivalent to psychiatric symptoms, behavioural syndromes as the same as psychiatric syndromes, and behavioural disorders as the same as psychiatric disorders.

It is well recognized that paediatricians manage a large proportion of childhood mental health problems (28). In this section we discuss situations where behavioural symptoms indicate the possible presence of particular psychiatric syndromes.

It is incorrect to assume without adequate assessment that the behaviour is due to the underlying developmental condition (see 'diagnostic overshadowing' below). Similarly, it is important to appreciate that mental health conditions in children with developmental disorders may manifest in atypical ways (see 'pathoplastic effects' in the section Assessment and diagnostic formulation below).

Mental health disorders often present as change, or deterioration, in the pattern of behaviour and/or function typical for that child. The presence of disordered behaviours or altered emotion, however, does not constitute a diagnosis. Three conditions are necessary to diagnose a mental disorder

- There must be persisting symptoms of disturbed behaviours or emotions which are abnormal in quality or quantity;

- The symptoms must cause distress or suffering to the individual or those around them; and

- The symptoms must cause some impairment of function. That is, they prevent the child from functioning at the level at which they would without the symptoms.

A general description of mental disorders affecting children and adolescents may be found in standard texts of child psychiatry. A clinically oriented source which paediatricians will find readable is the reference (29). In this section, we restrict discussion to aspects of mental health problems which are of particular relevance to children with developmental disabilities.

Assessment and diagnostic formulation

Could the behaviour be the symptomatic presentation of a psychiatric syndrome? We suggest the paediatrician approach this question as they would with any other health problem. That is, the question: could the behaviour be due to psychosis or depression is no different in principle from the question: could the behaviour be due to epilepsy or constipation?

In Chapter 3, we introduced the term 'diagnostic overshadowing'. This term has been used to describe the tendency for clinicians to attribute incorrectly behaviour disturbances of children and adolescents with developmental disabilities to the developmental disability alone.

Consider, for example, an adolescent with Velocardiofacial syndrome (VCFS, 22q11.2 deletion). The behaviour phenotype of this disorder includes shyness and anxiety. However, the individual may develop increasing social anxiety, with an uncharacteristically odd manner and increasingly paranoid misinterpretation of social messages. This deterioration may be considered a worsening of VCFS anxiety. However, individuals with this condition are at risk (about 33% (30)) of developing psychosis, and these symptoms may indicate that a psychotic syndrome may have emerged.

The 'pathoplastic' effect of developmental disability on the expression of typical mental signs and symptoms means that the disability alters how the mental health problem is clinically expressed. This occurs particularly in the presence of cognitive and communication impairments, as well as sensory disturbances. Because of this effect, presence of the underlying mental health problem may not be considered.

An example is the depressed, non-verbal teenager. They are not able to describe their sad mood, and depression is necessarily inferred from non-verbal signs as described below. A somatic example is the non-verbal child with pain. This may be suspected by an unexplained increase in behavioural agitation.

Because of this pathoplastic effect, it has been recognized that standard diagnostic criteria such as DSM-5 and ICD-11 may not describe the presentation of symptoms well in this population. In response to this, specialized classification systems have been developed for use with children and adolescents with developmental disabilities and are especially useful for patients with significant communication difficulties.

One of these developed in the United Kingdom is the Diagnostic Criteria-Learning Disorders (DC-LD (31)), although this is oriented to adults. It is a version of the ICD. Another classification system is a modification of DSM developed in the United States, the Diagnostic Manual—Intellectual Disability, 2nd Edition (DSM-ID-2, (32)). Paediatricians may choose to consult these manuals if a precise diagnostic label is required when ICD or DSM criteria do not fit well with a patient with developmental disability. The DM-ID-2 also provides a detailed discussion of the full range of mental disorders as they are seen in people with intellectual disability.

Treating mental disorders in children with developmental disabilities

In general

- Therapies requiring language skills are generally likely to be less available than non-verbal therapy such as play therapy.

- Therapies are more likely to be successful when directed towards building parent competency than direct work with the child.

- Non-verbal materials such as social stories in pictures can be useful, for example books by Sheila Hollins et al. are written for people with limited verbal abilities, addressing bereavement, being a victim of abuse, healthcare, and other issues; https://www.booksbeyondwords.co.uk/sheila-hollins.

- Responses to psychotropic medications are different when used in people with brain dysfunction. Side effects are more common. Children may be more sensitive and require doses lower than standard. See Chapter 5 for more information about this.

- In children with ID, therapies need to be appropriate for mental age, not chronological age.

Delirium

Key behaviours—Delirium

Behaviours that change as consciousness fluctuates over hours, including confusion and disorientation.

Delirium is a confusional syndrome reflecting an acute encephalopathy. This disturbance can be caused by any pathological process such as sepsis, metabolic disturbance, or drug toxicity. The result is relatively rapid and widespread brain dysfunction. Typically, there is a fluctuating level of consciousness with disorientation in time and or place. Visual hallucinations are a classical symptom.

The significance for children with developmental disabilities is:

1. A child with a brain which already has chronic dysfunction is more vulnerable to toxic brain processes.

2. If the child has limited communication, they may not communicate medical symptoms in an appropriate or timely manner.

3. If the child has limited communication, the confusional state may be less obvious.

Treatment is primarily to address the cause of the brain toxicity, but sedation, usually with antipsychotics, may be needed for symptomatic management whilst the cause of delirium is being investigated and addressed.

Psychosis

> # Key behaviours—Psychosis
>
> Unusual, unexpected behaviours arising from hallucinations, delusions, and thought disorder.

Syndromes of psychosis are seen with increased frequency among adolescents with developmental disabilities, particularly intellectual disabilities. This is presumably because underlying organic brain dysfunction is a likely vulnerability factor. Around 4% to 5% of intellectually disabled adults have been found to have schizophrenia (33), a rate ten times higher than the general population.

Psychosis is a syndrome seen in several disorders. Schizophrenia is a chronic psychosis accompanied by a decline in overall function, usually but not always commencing in later adolescence. The term 'schizoaffective disorder' is sometimes used when psychosis is accompanied by marked mood changes. If psychosis is a consequence of drug ingestion, the term 'Substance/Medication-Induced Psychotic Disorder' is used in DSM-5.

The cardinal symptoms or signs of psychosis are hallucinations, delusions, or thought disorder:

◆ Hallucinations are defined as a sensory (e.g. visual, auditory) perception in the absence of a causal sensory stimulus.

◆ Delusions are defined as fixed false beliefs which cannot be true and are inconsistent with the individual's culture.

◆ Thought disorder refers to disorders of thinking as judged by how it is expressed. These symptoms include but are not limited to: poverty of content of speech, pressure of speech, derailment, tangential thinking, incoherence, neologisms, word approximations, circumstantiality, loss of goal.

There is evidence that psychosis is over-diagnosed with individuals who have ID (34). This may derive, in part at least, from misdiagnosis of hallucinations. As an example, carers of an adolescent with developmental disability may observe the individual conducting conversations with absent persons or admitting to hearing voices of absent persons. However, if the paediatrician spends sufficient time questioning and observing the patient, it may become apparent that the individual is remembering conversations or just thinking about them out loud, rather than perceiving them without stimulus. Such memories often centre on troubling relationships or events in the individual's life, and the adolescent has no difficulty in distinguishing between the remembered conversations and current reality. Conversations with absent persons may be a socially inappropriate behaviour but they do not of themselves constitute hallucinations.

Similar caution needs to be exercised in the assessment of possible delusions. For example, carers may report that an individual with ID is unjustifiably complaining that adults or peers are saying hostile or critical things about them. It should be remembered that young people with disabilities experience a good deal of criticism, devaluation, mockery, and rejection. It is not surprising that some individuals develop a sensitivity to communications from others which could be interpreted as critical.

A patient, non-threatening interview will often reveal that the individual has not understood what was said by others. The 'persecutory' ideas may resolve with explanation. It is more common for individuals with developmental disabilities to be sensitive to perceived criticism, and sensitized from past criticism, than it is for them to experience true persecutory delusions.

Where delusions or hallucinations are truly present, the sophistication of their content correlates with developmental capacity. A 17-year-old with an IQ of 50 will not, for example, state that foreign spies are reading his mind via satellite. He may, however, believe that the people on the buses that go past his house are trying to harm him.

The unfortunate consequence of inaccurate diagnosis of psychotic illness is the over-prescription of antipsychotics. This leads to unnecessary sedation, impairment of adaptive function and long-term risk of tardive dyskinesia.

Obsessions and Obsessive-Compulsive Disorder

> ## Key behaviours: Obsessive-Compulsive Disorder
>
> Conversation characterized by obsessions (recurrent thought) with associated behavioural compulsions, either or both to a degree that is harmful for the child.

For children with developmental disorders, it may be difficult to distinguish preoccupations and rituals associated with their condition (particularly ASD) from the true obsessions of OCD.

According to the American Psychological Association,[2] obsessions are 'a persistent thought, idea, image, or impulse that is experienced as intrusive or inappropriate and results in marked anxiety, distress, or discomfort. Obsessions are often described as **ego-dystonic**,[3] in that they are experienced as alien or inconsistent with oneself and outside one's control (though this is not necessarily the case in children).' Compulsions are the motor form of obsessions, manifesting as repetitive actions.

Regarding obsessions, the interpretation text of DSM-5 notes that '[t]he individual attempts to ignore or suppress such thoughts, urges, or images, or to neutralise them with some other thought or action (i.e., by performing a compulsion)'.

The text of DSM5 further explains: 'The behaviours or mental acts are aimed at preventing or reducing anxiety or distress, or preventing some dreaded event or situation; however, these behaviours or mental acts are not connected in a realistic way with what they are designed to neutralize or prevent or are clearly excessive. Young children may not be able to articulate the aims of these behaviours or mental acts.'

The term 'obsessions' is commonly applied to the preoccupations seen in autism, Prader–Willi syndrome, and other developmental disorders, particularly those with frontal lobe impairments. Children and adolescents with these conditions commonly do not experience their obsessions or compulsions as egodystonic. They do not try to suppress them. They are not clearly intended to prevent a dreaded situation. For these reasons, these phenomena are usually

---

[2] American Psychological Association. https://dictionary.apa.org/obsession.

[3] American Psychological Association. https://dictionary.apa.org/ego-dystonic.

not true obsessions. Such thoughts are better characterized as **preoccupations** and the motor acts characterized as **rituals**.

A commonly associated concept is 'perseveration' in which the child's ideation is problematically fixated on an object or idea and is unable to shift from the item. This needs to be differentiated from wilful persistence. An example of wilful persistence is the child who repeatedly demands to have some request met, to the point where others find it annoying. It is a behaviour under the child's control. By contrast, true obsessions and preoccupations are not within the child's control or are very difficult for the child to control.

True OCD may occur in children with mild levels of ID.

Anti-anxiety medications are useful for both OCD and preoccupations and rituals. The use of anti-anxiety medications in autism to treat preoccupations has been discussed in the section on autism above.

For OCD, clomipramine is generally considered the most potent pharmacological treatment, however rates of problematic anticholinergic side effects are higher than the SSRIs. Cognitive-behavioural treatment (CBT) for children with OCD has benefit comparable to pharmacotherapy (35). Both may work together, with successful medical treatment enabling successful CBT. For the child, successful CBT requires an appropriate level of ownership, motivation, and capacity.

Depression

Key behaviours: Depression

In addition to reported alteration of mood, the following behaviours are observable:

- Sustained change from baseline

- Reduction in activities, participation, motivation

- Alteration of sleep and appetite

Depression can lead to withdrawal but can also lead to episodes of agitation, aggression, and worsening of stereotypic behaviours.

Depressive illness may occur in all individuals with developmental disorders, including those with the most severe intellectual disability. It is likely that clinically significant depression is commonly unrecognized, and under-diagnosed. That is because the cardinal symptoms of affective illness are based on self-reported mood states and experiences.

The ability both to conceptualize and report mood states varies with level of mental age and intellectual function. Adolescents with mild ID may be able to report mood states clearly.

Behaviours observable by parents, carers, teachers, and others include:

- Change in overall activity level (recent psychomotor retardation)
- Diurnal changes in activity and early morning waking.
- Weight loss
- A persisting sad facial expression
- Diminished pleasure in activities that were previously enjoyed, particularly social
- Increased stereotypic behaviour

Depressed mood can also be present in the context of Adjustment Disorders. This term describes a psychological response to a recognizable stressor but where the response is considered both problematic and excessive in severity or duration.

Management of depression usually requires a multimodal approach as determined by analysis of all contributing factors. Strategies include medications, psychotherapies both individual and family, and environmental approaches. These have been described in Chapter 5.

In monitoring the success of interventions, it is wise to assess mood level regularly. An example system is a 1 to 10 scale with 1 being the lowest mood the child can conceive, and 10 is normal happy mood. Mood can be monitored daily, or a couple of times per week, for example a school day and a weekend day. If the child's disability or mental age is such that they cannot rate their mood, parents/carers should be asked to rate their view of the child's mood based on its behavioural expression.

In addition to monitoring mood, we recommend a parallel assessment of function. This means rating the level of the child's participation in activities the child previously enjoyed.

Bipolar disorder and mood instability

Key behaviours of mania

- Time course is episodic
- Increased energy, decreased need for sleep

- Increased activity, for example talking, motor activity
- If the adolescent has enough language, there may be grandiosity
- Impaired/impulsive judgement

Bipolar disorder has been a controversial diagnosis in childhood (36, 37). It is now understood that it occurs far less frequently in the paediatric population than depression. True bipolar disorder in childhood or adolescence nearly always occurs where there is a strong family history of bipolar disorder.

Mania or hypomania occurs episodically. Where these symptoms are caused by a drug or other substance, the diagnosis made is Substance-/Medication-Induced Bipolar and Related Disorder. There are two relatively common situations in which this occurs in the paediatric population. One is as a consequence of stimulant use in some children, either prescribed for ADHD or used illicitly. The other is as an activating side effect of SSRI use, particularly fluoxetine (38).

More common in children with developmental disabilities is mood instability. This manifests as frequent fluctuation between hypomanic excitement and depressive withdrawal. This is presumably an expression of impaired function of the brain system which maintains a stable mood. Mood stabilizers may be trialled. A description of these is given in Chapter 5.

Disruptive Mood Dysregulation Disorder

Key behaviours: Disruptive Mood Dysregulation Disorder

Typical behaviours include severe recurrent temper outbursts out of proportion to the situation or provocation. Intervening mood is predominantly irritable or angry.

In DSM-5, a new disorder was added, Disruptive Mood Dysregulation Disorder (DMDD). It is described as the presentation of children with persistent irritability and frequent episodes of extreme behavioural dyscontrol in children up to 12 years of age.

These disorders have been demonstrated in research to be so frequently comorbid, especially in children with autism, that it is questionable whether the distinction between them is valid (37). For both, diagnosis needs to be considered in the context of developmental age and capacity rather than chronological age. Our clinical recommendation is to reserve the DMDD diagnosis for children where sad or depressed mood forms part of the picture.

Oppositional Defiant Disorder

> ### Key behaviours: Oppositional Defiant Disorder
>
> Developmentally inappropriate and problematically sustained angry and irritable mood in conjunction with refusal to cooperate and comply

Oppositional Defiant Disorder (ODD) is defined by a combination of mood and behaviour that are problematic for the child as well as those who have to manage them. It is likely that this cluster of symptoms arises from different causal processes in different children. The clinical picture of ODD co-occurs with developmental disorders such as ASD (39) and ADHD (40).

Consideration of ODD must be undertaken in developmental context. Rather than chronological age, behaviours are necessarily considered against developmental age-equivalent, particularly social age. A 9-year-old child with mild ID, for example, may have a developmental social age still in the preschool range.

In addition to the behavioural challenge of ODD, the diagnosis is significant because of prognostic implications. Whilst some children may 'grow out' of the clinical picture as they mature, for others the problems persist, potentially through adult life (41). For this reason, management should address the underlying cause as much as possible in addition to the resulting behaviours.

Suicidality

Suicidal thinking is more common in children whose lives are difficult due, but not restricted to their developmental disorder, where these children have capacity to reflect on their situation and see no way out of their predicament. Suicidal ideation is more common in children with ADHD (42) and specific reading disorders (43). Adolescents with mild intellectual disabilities may express suicidal ideation (44).

The challenge for paediatricians is to consider the possibility of such thinking. This begins with an understanding of what life is like for the child, and a relationship of trust that enables them to discuss their thoughts. Suicide risk assessment involves a mix of open ended (e.g. how are you feeling) and specific questions (45) such as:

◆ Have you thought about hurting yourself?

◆ How often do you think about this?

◆ Do you have a plan?

◆ Have you tried to end your life? How recently?

If the risk is significant, this requires a decisive and generally immediate response. If the level of risk is uncertain, seeking a timely second opinion from mental health professionals is recommended.

Anxiety

Anxiety may be considered a psychological disturbance leading to impairment and distress when it is:

◆ **Too much:** The anxiety experienced is excessive for the level of threat, and causing problems for the child.

◆ **Too little:** Anxiety may be pathologically deficient in some children with conduct disorder. Children with disturbed attachment may demonstrate a pathological lack of stranger anxiety.

With anxiety generally:

◆ Biologically based vulnerability to anxiety problems has a strong genetic component. In addition, response to anti-anxiety medications is typically consistent across generations.

◆ A commonly used and helpful scale to measure anxiety is the Spence Children's Anxiety Scale.[4] There is a literature on its use in children with autism (46).

◆ The presence of anxiety in one form, such as generalized anxiety, increases the risk of anxiety of another type. An exception is Williams syndrome, where high levels of phobic anxiety co-occur with low levels of stranger anxiety.

If anxiety is a problem for a child it is necessary to describe it further. Just concluding a child has a problem with anxiety is insufficient to guide intervention.

---

[4] https://www.scaswebsite.com/.

Types of anxiety disorders

Key symptoms described below are quoted from, or refer to, DSM-5 criteria (47).

Separation anxiety disorder

Developmentally inappropriate, problematic and excessive fear or anxiety concerning separation from those to whom the individual is primarily attached.

The term 'developmentally inappropriate' is important. We have seen children for example aged 10 with severe ID and a mental age of 3 who want to sleep in the parents' bed labelled as having separation anxiety disorder. It is normal for a 3-year-old to want to sleep in the parents' bed.

Selective mutism

This is marked by consistent failure to speak in specific social situations in which there is an expectation for speaking (e.g. at school) despite speaking in other situations. This is to the degree that is harmful for the child.

Selective mutism is not a form of autistic social communication impairment. It could be considered the opposite where children are over-sensitive to social context. In selective mutism, the child chooses not to speak, despite being capable of doing so. In autistic social communication impairments, the child is unable to communicate normally.

In addition to the contribution of anxiety to mute behaviour selectively, the child may have a degree of underlying language disorder (48), choosing not to talk because it is hard for them as well as socially stressful.

Management is a combination of (1) reducing anxiety, (2) supporting language, and (3) behavioural incentives to break the habit of staying quiet.

Specific phobia

Behaviours specific to a particular object or challenge that arise from fear/anxiety.

The anxiety may be expressed in behaviours typical of the child's developmental age, for example crying, tantrums, freezing or clinging. A specific phobia (e.g. dogs) may arise as a response to past trauma.

Social anxiety disorder

Marked fear or anxiety about one or more social situations in which the individual is exposed to possible scrutiny by others.

Example situations include social interactions (e.g. having a conversation, meeting unfamiliar people), being observed (e.g. eating or drinking), and performing in front of others (e.g. giving a speech).

For children, social anxiety must occur in peer settings and not just during interactions with adults. Performance anxiety is one pattern in which the child cannot participate in group activities because of intense fear that their performance will be denigrated by others. This is more likely when a child with a disability has been teased.

Panic disorder

A panic attack is an abrupt surge of intense fear or intense discomfort that reaches a peak within minutes. How this is expressed varies with the individual but typically is characterized by flight or freeze. Panic disorder is recurrent unexpected panic attacks.

The fear is accompanied by particular symptoms and behaviour described in DSM-5, such as sweating, palpitations, and trembling. These are the physiological and behavioural consequences of a sudden increase in adrenaline and sympathetic nervous system discharge.

Agoraphobia

The behaviours of agoraphobia arise from heightened fear or anxiety about two (or more) of the following five situations:

1. Using public transportation (e.g. automobiles, buses, trains, ships, planes).

2. Being in open spaces (e.g. parking lots, market places, bridges).

3. Being in enclosed places (e.g. shops, theatres, cinemas).

4. Standing in line or being in a crowd.

5. Being outside of the home alone.

Generalized Anxiety Disorder

Generalized anxiety disorder (GAD) is a sustained, developmentally inappropriate, and excessive anxiety and worry (apprehensive expectation) across a range of contexts or situations that causes harm to the child. Its behavioural expression varies with these contexts and situations as well as how the individual child behaves in response to this anxiety and worry.

Pharmacological treatment of anxiety problems

SSRIs and mirtazapine are generally effective anti-anxiety agents. Their use is described above in Chapter 5. Moclobemide is safe but probably less effective. Hydroxyzine is an antihistamine used quite frequently in the United States for treatment of anxiety disorders but there is limited evidence of effectiveness.

Psychological treatment of anxiety problems

A wide variety of psychological approaches have been utilized in the treatment of anxiety in childhood. The paediatrician has an important role in selecting children for whom these strategies may be effective. For success, children must be able to understand the concepts, along with the capacity and motivation to undertake the therapeutic activities. What they learn in an office setting is only useful if they are able to use it in everyday life.

The most common strategies with good evidence include Cognitive-Behavioural Therapy (49). Acceptance and Commitment-based therapy may be a gentle strategy with similar efficacy (50). Online psychological therapies are also available (51). The combination of pharmacological and psychological treatments is superior to either alone (52).

Trauma- and stressor-related disorders

> # Key behaviours: Trauma and stress
>
> Behavioural responses disproportionate to the presumed level of actual threat in situations. These are generally the behavioural expression of disproportionate emotional responses to these situations.

Threat includes social situations (e.g. fear of making others unhappy, abandonment) for children with attachment disorders as well as threat of possible hurt (e.g. raised voices) for children who have experienced trauma.

General issues of threat and emotional responses were discussed in Chapter 2. Children generally are at risk from trauma, stress, and abuse because of their size, maturity, understanding, and capacity to defend themselves. Children with developmental disorders are at higher risk. They are likely to be less able to defend themselves and less able to understand others' behaviour. Around 25% of children with disabilities experience violence and abuse (53).

Current stresses

> # Practice tip: Is the child's stress due to current circumstances?
>
> Current stresses and traumas need to be addressed before trying to modify behaviours resulting from the stress. Attempts to modify behaviour while threat is ongoing will not succeed

Possible current problems include:

- Demands that the child cannot manage, coupled with punitive responses based on incorrect attribution (e.g. the child is not trying hard enough).

- Bullying and other forms of devaluation.

- Abuse (physical, sexual, emotional).

- Environmental threat (domestic violence, unsafe neighbourhoods, war).

Recent stresses

Recent problems mean the stress is no longer occurring, but its consequences persist.

Acute distress disorder

This describes a severe psychological decompensation occurring in the period 3 days to 1 month after a life-threatening experience.

Adjustment disorder

Adjustment disorders are excessively distressing and disabling psychological symptoms occurring within 3 months of the stressor and lasting less than 6 months. The symptoms are depressed mood and/or anxiety and/or disturbance of conduct.

Past problems

The DSM-5 includes four disorders in this group:

Reactive Attachment Disorder

Reactive Attachment Disorder (RAD) is one form of consequence of deprivation or abuse. The early childhood experience encodes a predictive belief that they cannot show normal trust. This is most evident with people on whom the child most depends.

Behaviours arising from this disordered capacity to trust have many forms. These include:

- The child rarely or minimally seeks comfort when distressed and minimally responds to comfort when distressed.

- The child whose behaviour serves to test boundaries, on a persistent basis, experienced by the caregiver as an irresolvable test of consistency and care.

- The child whose behaviour in relationships varies unpredictably from intimate and engaged to angry and distrusting.

If ongoing attachment disorder is likely, the paediatrician can usefully help care-givers understand that this behaviour is not a reflection of the quality of their care but is instead a biologically encoded set of beliefs and responses unrelated to their care. RAD typically takes years to resolve, even with the best care and treatment.

Disinhibited social engagement disorder

This pattern of behaviour occurs as a consequence of early childhood abuse or deprivation. It has been considered a variation of attachment disorder. The central feature of this condition is that the child has a pathological lack of stranger anxiety, tending to wander away from caregivers or engage in overly familiar physical behaviour with unfamiliar adults.

Management has the goal of embedding self-protective behaviours at a habituation level.

Post-traumatic Stress Disorder (PTSD)

In PTSD, trauma is experienced as an overwhelming threat and recorded in memory as such. Symptoms of PTSD are one or more of:

- Recurrent, involuntary, and intrusive distressing memories or dreams of the traumatic event(s).

- Dissociative reactions (e.g. flashbacks)

- Distress and physiological reactions if exposed to cues that resemble the trauma.

- Avoidance of stimuli that remind the individual of the trauma.

- Impaired cognition and mood in association with recollection of the trauma.

- Alterations in arousal and reactivity beginning after the events.

- Duration of the disturbance for more than 1 month.

Complex PTSD extends beyond episodic triggered patterns of response to include persisting changes to an individual's baseline emotional and psychological state. It is particularly relevant for children exposed to prolonged abuse. Complex PTSD is described in ICD-11 as meeting all the diagnostic requirements for PTSD, and additionally, severe and persistent:

1. problems in affect regulation;

2. beliefs about oneself as diminished, defeated, or worthless, accompanied by feelings of shame, guilt, or failure related to the traumatic event; and

3. difficulties in sustaining relationships and in feeling close to others. These symptoms cause significant impairment in personal, family, social, educational, occupational, or other important areas of functioning.

In all the above trauma-related disorders, the paediatrician has a role in:

◆ Identifying stress in the child's life: current, recent, and past.

◆ Reducing sources of current stress as possible.

◆ Educating parents, particularly if they feel responsible for the child's on-going struggles.

◆ Supporting parents in the long term.

◆ Discouraging ineffective treatments.

◆ Advocating for continuity of support for carers.

◆ Judicious use of supportive pharmacotherapy.

Ingestion and elimination disorders

Feeding-related disorders

Pica

Pica is the eating of non-nutritive or non-food substances. Pica is seen in a number of genetic developmental disabilities involving hyperphagia, especially Prader–Willi and SchaafYang syndromes and Cri du Chat syndrome (54). Pica is seen in individuals with severe ID.

Pica is associated with nutritional deficiencies of iron and zinc, though the direction of causality is unclear, since supplementation with these minerals has not corrected the pica (55). The motivations for pica may remain unclear.

Treatment for pica usually proceeds on behavioural lines derived from functional assessment (see Chapter 5). An SSRI may be indicated in an attempt to reduce the anxiety forces driving obsessional elements in the behaviour.

Rumination disorder

Rumination is the repeated regurgitation and rechewing of food in the absence of organic gastrointestinal pathology. It is not associated with nausea. Rumination can cause weight loss and dehydration.

Rumination in children with intellectual disabilities does not appear to be dependent on social interaction but rather by autonomous sensory reward. Behavioural strategies can be effective, with satiation having good evidence (56). Satiation involves providing larger food portions or higher calorie foods.

Avoidant/Restrictive Food Intake Disorder

In DSM-5, Avoidant/Restrictive Food Intake Disorder (ARFID) is exemplified by apparent lack of interest in food or avoidance of food sufficient to cause inadequate nutrition.

Peculiarities of food preference or insistence are common in autism and are discussed above (Autism: Restricted diet, avoidant/restrictive food intake disorder (ARFID)).

In other children, more resistant and problematic symptoms may require input from an occupational therapist, psychologist or dietitian with specialized interest in this area.

Elimination disorders

Elimination disorders are those associated with defaecation and urination. As with all the challenges discussed in this section, these are likely to be associated with other problem behaviours and occur more commonly in children who have developmental disability. A useful resource is the work of von Gontard and colleagues.[5]

Enuresis

Enuresis is involuntary urination at night, a developmentally defined condition as night-time continence is an acquired skill. There is often a strong family history. This problem is commonly seen in paediatric practice.

Developmental disorders, by definition, impact child development over time. This may include the capacity to learn continence during the night. Understanding and management of enuresis is necessarily undertaken in a developmental context.

Enuresis itself is not a behavioural disorder. It can increase the likelihood of difficult behaviour if the child feels shame, is subject to expectations they cannot manage, or experiences punishment and abuse for this problem. As with encopresis (the repeated, involuntary or voluntary, passing of stool in inappropriate places), however, it is a problem that may be dealt with more easily, with positive impact on child behaviour and self-esteem.

In these cases, the paediatrician has an important role in reviewing how the enuresis is currently managed. Behavioural strategy (e.g. using enuresis alarms)

---

[5] Von Gontard A, Neveus T.https://www.mackeith.co.uk/book/management-of-disorders-of-bladder-and-bowel-control-in-childhood/. Mac Keith Press. Published January 2006. Accessed 10/04/2025.

requires a level of capacity and motivation from the child. Pharmacotherapy is effective, particularly the situational use of desmopressin. In addition to symptom supports, it is important to consider the psychological health of the child. They need to understand that enuresis is not their fault and beyond their control, and be supported in living with this.

Encopresis

For children with ID, mild to severe ASD, and CP, learning faecal continence may require explicit, stepwise, and repetitive behavioural training to both establish and maintain this functional skill.

Persisting soiling may be an indicator of abuse. Encopresis most commonly occurs in the presence of cyclic constipation/overflow. Management with bowel emptying and ensuring soft stools are passed regularly is still necessary. For children who have developmental disorders, ensuring daily stool passage and recordings of stool consistency for longer periods than usual may be needed.

A child may fear shame from faecal leakage they cannot detect or control. Their behaviour reflects how they manage this risk. Faecal soiling is a common reason for bullying. Alongside managing the soiling, the paediatrician should consider the child's experience, managed if necessary.

Management of soiling is a priority. If the child feels safer with regards to bowel control, other problems are likely to be managed more easily. We suggest it be addressed early when problems are multiple and complex.

Smearing

Faecal smearing is a difficult problem to manage because it is aesthetically unpleasant. It occurs predominantly in children with ID but may occur when children are deeply disturbed for reasons such as abuse/trauma and more severe mental health conditions.

The first stage of paediatric management is to exclude organic drivers for this behaviour. These may include irritation (e.g. intestinal worms), pain from recurrent constipation, or physiological complications such as tears, fissures, and prolapse.

In the absence of correctable pathology, management depends on the hypothesis of causation. Example hypotheses include:

- The child experiences secondary gain. This behaviour triggers a response from caregivers that provides incentive to maintain the behaviour.

- The child is neglected, self-stimulating in the presence of social deprivation.

- The child for some reason gains pleasure from the smell/texture of the experience.

Assessment using the tools described in Chapter 3, ABC analysis and analysis of contextual variation are required to generate hypotheses about the cause.

The simplest intervention is to prevent access. This may include, for example, wearing nappies (diapers) underneath full body clothing that the child cannot readily remove.

Associated with prevention of access, Differential Reinforcement of Other Behaviours (DRO) (see Chapter 5) is useful. An example alternative behaviour is playing with material that has similar texture, such as playdough mixed with strong-smelling materials that the child likes, (e.g. ground spices).

Somatic and conversion disorders

Recurrent abdominal pain

Recurrent abdominal pain is relatively common in children. In the sequence of excluding organic causes, a point is reached where further investigations are no longer of sufficient benefit compared to risk. In such cases, the challenge is to manage the child's expectations, capacity to self-care, and related family behaviour. Towards these goals the following principles may be helpful:

Working with the child and family regarding the pain should include the following considerations:

- The pain experienced by the child is real;

- The probability of serious organic pathology has been excluded. Further investigation is likely to cause more harm than the pain itself, and not likely to find a significant, treatable cause.

- Management may involve courage, distraction, general health (eating, exercise, sleep), such that the child is rewarded for 'how well' they adapt to their circumstances.

In finding and managing sources of stress, keep in mind:

- Recurrent abdominal pain may be the presentation of significant problems within the family. Formal family therapy may be necessary before stress is reduced to the degree that the child's pain is able to settle.

- Other potential sources of stress include problems at school (e.g. learning problems, bullying).

Psychogenic Non-epileptic Seizures (PNES)

According to Kozlowska et al. (57), psychogenic non-epileptic seizures 'collect together a range of atypical neurophysiological responses to emotional distress, physiological stressors and danger', which mimic epileptic seizures. The episodes may be grouped according to the physiological mechanism involved. These authors describe these groups as

1. Dissociative PNES

2. Triggered dissociative PNES, triggers including:

   ○ Hyperventilation

   ○ Vocal cord adduction

   ○ Activation from the Valsalva manoeuvre

   ○ Reflex activation of the vagus

3. Hypomobility defence responses similar to paralysis from fear, presenting as PNES

The diagnosis of PNES is likely to be more acceptable when it is explained as a response to psychological stress, with demonstrable intervening physiological mechanisms.

To manage these, children can be trained to increase their heart rate variability with slow breathing. An example tool to help them is the MyCalmBeat app (58). This process can be effective in preventing progress to PNES. Further details of this intervention are given in an adjacent paper by Kozlowska et al. (59).

In children with cognitive impairments, PNES is thought to occur more often in response to immediate environmental triggers and be more dependent on reinforcement. Thus, there is a greater reliance on environmental manipulation as part of treatment. This pattern will be more readily determined if a behavioural diary is kept for a month or so, including the behaviour, time and place circumstances, antecedents (precipitating), and consequences (perpetuating, palliating).

Other conversion disorders are managed similarly to recurrent abdominal pain and PNES.

Chapter summary

For children with behaviour problems in the context of developmental disorders it is useful to determine the extent to which the behaviour:

◆ Is a direct consequence of the developmental disorder/syndrome;

◆ Is related both to the condition and how it is managed; or

◆ Not a direct consequence of the condition, arising primarily for other, usually individual, reasons.

In this chapter we discuss specific conditions. Where the behaviour arises as part of the diagnosis/syndrome itself, condition-specific research is likely to provide information regarding management options.

Appendix 6. 1—Selected syndromes with 'behavioural phenotypes'

The following syndromes have been chosen as they are commonly seen in paediatric practice.

Down syndrome

Behaviour

- Relatively low levels of behaviour problems compared with other causes of ID.

- Early onset of Alzheimer-type dementia (average 50 years, but sometimes earlier).

- Behaviour may change due to 'unexplained functional regression' (60).

- Behavioural consequences of low thyroid function.

Cognitive features

- ID (mild to severe).

Clinical considerations

- Check for depression (try SSRI medications).

- Treat hypothyroidism if present.

- Check for conductive hearing loss.

Fragile X syndrome

Behaviour

- Initial social anxiety with aversion to eye contact. Mostly Fragile X people can become friendly with familiarity.

- Stereotypies, hand flapping, hand biting, notably with anxiety or excitement.

- Some meet criteria for ASD in childhood with associated behaviours.

Cognitive features

- Boys' mild to moderate ID.

- Girls—two-thirds average range, one-third mild ID.

- Often decline in measured IQ through childhood.

Clinical considerations

- SSRI medications can help anxiety.

Prader–Willi syndrome (PWS)

Behaviour

- Severe hyperphagia, including pica.

- Severe temper tantrums, disproportionate escalation when thwarted.

- Pain insensitivity leading to behaviours such as skin picking, rectal gouging.

- Hypersomnolence.

- Obsessional behaviours, commonly including hoarding and repetitive questioning.

- Intermittent psychosis behaviour. Risk of psychosis is greater in those with the uniparental disotomy (UPD) cause compared with those with a deletion cause for PWS (61).

Cognitive features

- Typically, mild ID, occasionally moderate ID or normal range IQ.

- Emotional maturity less developed than intellectual level.

Clinical considerations

- Behaviour interventions towards strict, regular, rules-based expectations and opportunities to eat.

- Medication treatment or eating behaviour has not led to consistent patterns of results (62). Newer treatments such as GLP-1 receptor agonist medications may be effective (63).

- Medical treatments, such as growth hormone in childhood, management of sleep disturbance.

Angelman syndrome

Behaviour

- Heightened levels of laughing and smiling, a happy demeanour, excessive sociability, aggression, impulsivity, and sleep disorders (64).

- Fascination for water, hand flapping, self-injury.

- Disturbed sleep.

Cognitive features

- Severe to profound ID.

Clinical considerations

- Gastroesophageal reflux requires treatment, as do sleep problems and seizures.

22q11 (Velocardiofacial syndrome)

Behaviour

- Shy, anxious.

- Increased risk of schizophrenia-like psychosis.

Cognitive features

- Usually mild ID, sometimes average IQ.

Clinical considerations

- SSRIs for anxiety, antipsychotics for psychosis.

Williams syndrome

Behaviour

- Hyperacusis, behaviours in response to overwhelming sound.

- High phobic anxiety.

- Problematically low level of social anxiety, indiscriminately friendly behaviour.

Cognitive features

- Low mild to moderate ID.

- Expressive language is better than receptive language, and language skills are generally higher than non-verbal conceptual skills.

Clinical considerations

- Recognize that comprehension may be lower than spoken language implies.

- Medical management of anxiety-related problems.

- Protect girls from sexual exploitation.

Tuberous Sclerosis Complex

Behaviour

- Behaviours arising from mood/anxiety disturbance, aggression, and tantrums.

- ADHD behaviours, such as hyperactive and impulsive.

- Disturbed self-regulation, sleep/eating.

- Behaviours arising from low social understanding, including autism-related behaviours.

Cognitive features

- Variable levels of ID in about 50% of cases.

- Child-specific neurocognitive problems (e.g. executive and visuo-spatial deficits) may occur, requiring individual neuropsychological assessment.

Clinical considerations

- mTOR inhibitors are under trial.

- Otherwise, treatment according to neurodevelopmental consequences.

XO (Turner) syndrome

Behaviour

- Anxiety (with associated behaviour) is common as a primary trait as well as an adaptation to learning and social problems.

Cognitive features

◆ Overall intellectual function is generally in the normal range.

◆ Specific neurocognitive problems are common in non-verbal domains, including visual-spatial cognition, executive function, social cognition, and higher-order language comprehension.

Clinical considerations

◆ Recognition that comprehension may fall below language competency.

◆ Medical treatment of co-occurring ADHD and Anxiety.

◆ Active management of growth and endocrine function may benefit behaviour, mental health and cognitive capacity.

XXY (Klinefelter) and XYY syndrome

Behaviour

◆ Both carry risk of problem behaviour, possibly secondary to neurocognitive challenges.

◆ Traditional thinking has been that XXY is more internalizing (feminine) and XYY more externalizing (masculine). This is not likely to be true because of ascertainment biases.

Cognitive features

◆ IQ average for these conditions is lower than population mean. Many individuals have IQ in the normal range.

◆ Both syndromes carry risk for specific neurocognitive problems, such as with language, learning, and executive functions.

Clinical considerations

◆ Management of behaviour according to understanding of individual developmental competencies and temperament.

◆ Hormonal therapy may diminish risk of behaviour problems.

Smith Magenis syndrome (17p11.2 deletion)

Behaviour

◆ Intense anxiety across a range of anxiety domains. Symptoms of ADHD are common. Self-injury is characteristic.

- Reversal of sleep pattern: hypersomnolence during day and insomnia at night.

- Decreased pain sensitivity.

Cognitive features and clinical impact

- Mild to moderate ID.

- Distinct facial and cranial dysmorphology.

- Corpus Callosum abnormalities.

Clinical considerations

- Sleep problems are treated with melatonin receptor agonists, β1-adrenergic antagonists, and stimulant medications. Improved sleep management often brings about improved behaviour.

- Check for hearing impairment.

- Check for sources of pain as these may not be reported directly by the child but are expressed in behaviour disturbance.

Appendix 6.2—Cases

Case 1. Jack

Jack is a boy diagnosed with FASD and ADHD.

Discussion

How does an understanding of Jack's disability and condition inform your management of his difficult behaviour?

Causation: The diagnosis of FASD sends a clear message both of causation and consequence. In short, Jack has suffered brain damage. This message is critical if those working with him are to adopt a compassionate and supportive approach.

Complexity: The diagnosis of FASD is made when at least three significant neurological systems are impacted to a 2SD (two standard deviations below the mean) degree of impairment. That sends a message that the changes are not trivial and, equally importantly, they are coexisting. For Jack, this reduces his resilience options, with less that 'works' to fall back on. In FASD, the totality of impact is more than the sum of the parts.

What does the diagnosis mean for the longer term?

After intrauterine brain injury there is potential for neuroplastic rehabilitation, however this potential tapers with time. Jack is now 9 years old. It is reasonable to think he has potential to build competency, but to a limited degree. After he moves through puberty, this potential further reduces.

In the longer term this means that Jack has to learn how to 'live with' his impairments rather than overcome them. This is more than the management of problems such as behavioural episodes. This requires stable, future-oriented, regular longitudinal care from the paediatrician, all the way through to adult transition.

Case 2. Jade

Jade is a 14-year-old girl in her second year of high school.

Discussion

How does an understanding of her disability and condition inform your management of her behaviour problems?

For an intelligent, articulate child with ASD, there is a risk that her deeper impairment is overlooked and too much will be expected of her. Jade's diagnosis implies a fundamental problem with social intuition, perspective taking, and capacity to manage social behaviour.

Intelligence enables insight. Understanding she is different, isolated, and somewhat of a 'misfit' can challenge mental health. A second risk is that her surface behaviours mask the turmoil beneath.

For cases where a medical cause has been identified or hypothesized, how might this information alter your understanding and management of their behaviour?

It is unlikely a medical aetiology will be identified for Jade's ASD, however it is reasonable to assume her ASD has a genetic basis given her family history. At the age of 14 it is clear this is more than a 'developmental delay', likely to persist into and throughout adult life.

What does the diagnosis mean for the longer term?

In Jade's case there are impairments attributable to her ASD that she will have to deal with throughout her life. Her prognosis is not necessarily poor, however. Jade is likely to have the intelligence to learn how to manage her life's social challenges. With support and encouragement, she could well find vocational and social ecosystems where she fits in without unsustainable effort that play to her strengths.

To enjoy her life in this way, the lessons of her current situation are important. She needs to learn how to manage functional challenges without avoidance. She needs to learn how to manage social challenges without behavioural escalation. These competencies will benefit her throughout her life.

Case 3. Alfred

Alfred has Down syndrome with moderate ID.

Discussion

What specific risks does Down syndrome carry for problem behaviour? Where they are relevant to understanding and managing behaviour, how might you assess these?

The central risk is confusion leading to anxiety. The sociability of most children with Down syndrome potentially leads to a perception they understand more than they do. An easy approach to adjustment of expectations is to consider their developmental 'age equivalent' level of comprehension, and manage his behaviour at this level.

Not all children with Down syndrome are social. Meta-analysis suggests that 16% to 18% of children with Down syndrome have autism, and so this condition needs to be considered in evaluating his irritability and perseverative behaviours.

Other influences on behaviour include possible conductive hearing loss, hypothyroidism, seizures, and other health problems associated with Down syndrome. Alfred has a predisposition to impulse control problems, as evidenced by the family history of ADHD and substance use disorders. All these potential risks can be assessed in standard ways via history, examination, and additional medical investigations when necessary.

The genetic basis of Down syndrome is permanent. How do these risks and their impact on behaviour change over time, particularly looking into his teenage and adult years?

Alfred's trisomy 21 will last his entire life, but the manifestations of his genetic condition will change over time. He has the capacity to develop skills and adaptive behaviours like other children with developmental disabilities. As a teenager, he has made progress in language and cause-and-effect thinking, with more capacity to think first before acting impulsively. Cognitive decline and early onset of dementia is common in adults with Down syndrome over 40 years. In young adults with Down syndrome, cognitive decline would be more likely due to social isolation, lack of stimulation, and depression.

References

(1) Tan Q, Orsso CE, Deehan EC, Triador L, Field CJ, Tun HM, et al. Current and emerging therapies for managing hyperphagia and obesity in Prader–Willi syndrome: A narrative review. *Obes Rev.* 2020;21(5):e12992.

(2) Chapman M, Iddon P, Atkinson K, Brodie C, Mitchell D, Parvin G, et al. The misdiagnosis of epilepsy in people with intellectual disabilities: a systematic review. *Seizure.* 2011;20(2):101–106.

(3) Oluwabusi OO, Parke S, Ambrosini PJ. Tourette syndrome associated with attention deficit hyperactivity disorder: The impact of tics and psychopharmacological treatment options. *World J Clin Pediatr.* 2016;5(1):128–135.

(4) Hours C, Recasens C, Baleyte JM. ASD and ADHD comorbidity: What are we talking about? *Front Psychiatry.* 2022;13:837424.

(5) Joshi G, Wilens T, Firmin ES, Hoskova B, Biederman J. Pharmacotherapy of attention deficit/hyperactivity disorder in individuals with autism spectrum disorder: A systematic review of the literature. *J Psychopharmacol Oxf Engl.* 2021;35(3):203–10.

(6) Russell G, Stapley S, Newlove-Delgado T, Salmon A, White R, Warren F, et al. Time trends in autism diagnosis over 20 years: A UK population-based cohort study. *J Child Psychol Psychiatry.* 2022;63(6):674–82.

(7) Shaw KA, Williams S, Patrick ME, et al. Prevalence and Early Identification of Autism Spectrum Disorder Among Children Aged 4 and 8 Years—Autism and Developmental Disabilities Monitoring Network, 16 Sites, United States, 2022. *MMWR Surveill Summ.* 2025;74(No. SS-2):1–22. doi:http://dx.doi.org/10.15585/mmwr.ss7402a1

(8) Fombonne E. Editorial: Is autism overdiagnosed? *J Child Psychol Psychiatry.* 2023;64(5):711–714.

(9) Skellern C, Schluter P, McDowell M. From complexity to category: Responding to diagnostic uncertainties of autistic spectrum disorders. *J Paediatr Child Health.* 2005;41(8):407–412.

(10) Williams K, Brignell A, Randall M, Silove N, Hazell P. Selective serotonin reuptake inhibitors (SSRIs) for autism spectrum disorders (ASD). *Cochrane Database Syst Rev.* 2013;(8):CD004677.

(11) Einfeld SL, Piccinin AM, Mackinnon A, Hofer SM, Taffe J, Gray KM, et al. Psychopathology in young people with intellectual disability. *JAMA.* 2006;296(16):1981–1989.

(12) Thapar A, Pine DS, Leckman JF, Scott S, Snowling MJ, Taylor EA, eds. *Rutter's Child and Adolescent Psychiatry.* 6th ed. Wiley-Blackwell; 2015.

(13) Emerson E, Einfeld S, Stancliffe RJ. The mental health of young children with intellectual disabilities or borderline intellectual functioning. *Soc Psychiatry Psychiatr Epidemiol.* 2010;45(5):579–587.

(14) Emerson E, Einfeld S. Emotional and behavioural difficulties in young children with and without developmental delay: A bi-national perspective. *J Child Psychol Psychiatry.* 2010;51(5):583–593.

(15) McDowell M. Specific learning disability. *J Paediatr Child Health.* 2018;54(10): 1077–1083.

(16) Ng L, Karunasinghe N, Benjamin CS, Ferguson LR. Beyond PSA: Are new prostate cancer biomarkers of potential value to New Zealand doctors? *N Z Med J.* 2012;125(1353). Accessed April 15, 2020. https://www.nzma.org.nz/journal-articles/ beyond-psa-are-new-prostate-cancer-biomarkers-of-potential-value-to-new-zealand- doctors/

(17) Rogers M, Hwang H, Toplak M, Weiss M, Tannock R. Inattention, working memory, and academic achievement in adolescents referred for attention deficit/hyperactivity disorder (ADHD). *Child Neuropsychol J Norm Abnorm Dev Child Adolesc.* 2011;17(5):444–458.

(18) Andrén P, Jakubovski E, Murphy TL, Woitecki K, Tarnok Z, Zimmerman-Brenner S, et al. European clinical guidelines for Tourette syndrome and other tic disorders- version 2.0. Part II: Psychological interventions. *Eur Child Adolesc Psychiatry.* 2022;31(3):403–423.

(19) Müller-Vahl KR, Szejko N, Verdellen C, Roessner V, Hoekstra PJ, Hartmann A, et al. European clinical guidelines for Tourette syndrome and other tic disorders: Summary statement. *Eur Child Adolesc Psychiatry.* 2022;31(3):377–382.

(20) Deeb W, Malaty IA, Mathews CA. Tourette disorder and other tic disorders. *Handb Clin Neurol.* 2019;165:123–153.

(21) Rzepka-Migut B, Paprocka J. Efficacy and safety of melatonin treatment in children with autism spectrum disorder and attention-deficit/hyperactivity disorder—a review of the literature. *Brain Sci.* 2020;10(4):219.

(22) Yuge K, Nagamitsu S, Ishikawa Y, Hamada I, Takahashi H, Sugioka H, et al. Long-term melatonin treatment for the sleep problems and aberrant behaviors of children with neurodevelopmental disorders. *BMC Psychiatry.* 2020;20(1):445.

(23) Fetal alcohol spectrum disorders in Australia—the future is prevention. PHRP. 2015 https://www.phrp.com.au/issues/march-2015-volume-25-issue-2/fetal-alcohol-spect rum-disorders-in-australia-the-future-is-prevention/

(24) Kambeitz C, Klug MG, Greenmyer J, Popova S, Burd L. Association of adverse childhood experiences and neurodevelopmental disorders in people with fetal alcohol spectrum disorders (FASD) and non-FASD controls. *BMC Pediatr.* 2019;19(1):498.

(25) Caputo C, Wood E, Jabbour L. Impact of fetal alcohol exposure on body systems: A systematic review. *Birth Defects Res Part C Embryo Today Rev.* 2016;108(2):174–180.

(26) Rasmussen C, Andrew G, Zwaigenbaum L, Tough S. Neurobehavioural outcomes of children with fetal alcohol spectrum disorders: A Canadian perspective. *Paediatr Child Health.* 2008;13(3):185–191.

(27) Davis E, Saeed SA, Antonacci DJ. Anxiety disorders in persons with developmental disabilities: empirically informed diagnosis and treatment. Reviews literature on

anxiety disorders in DD population with practical take-home messages for the clinician. *Psychiatr Q.* 2008;79(3):249–263.

(28) Royal Australasian College of Physicians. The Role of Paediatricians in the Provision of Mental Health Services to Children and Young People. [Internet]. https://www.racp. edu.au/docs/default-source/advocacy-library/racp---the-role-of-paediatricians-in-the-provision-of-mental-health-services-to-children-and-young-people.pdf

(29) Goodman R, Scott S. *Child and Adolescent Psychiatry.* 3rd ed. Wiley-Blackwell; 2012.

(30) Gothelf D, Feinstein C, Thompson T, Gu E, Penniman L, Van Stone E, et al. Risk factors for the emergence of psychotic disorders in adolescents with 22q11.2 deletion syndrome. *Am J Psychiatry.* 2007;164(4):663–669.

(31) Szymanski LS. DC-LD (diagnostic criteria for psychiatric disorders for use with adults with learning disabilities/mental retardation). *J Intellect Disabil Res.* 2002;46(6):525–527.

(32) Fletcher RJ, Barnhill J, Cooper SA, eds. *DM-ID-2: Diagnostic Manual, Intellectual Disability: A Textbook of Diagnosis of Mental Disorders in Persons with Intellectual Disability.* 2nd ed. NADD Press; 2018.

(33) Morgan VA, Leonard H, Bourke J, Jablensky A. Intellectual disability co-occurring with schizophrenia and other psychiatric illness: population-based study. *Br J Psychiatry J Ment Sci.* 2008;193(5):364–372.

(34) McLaren JL, Lichtenstein JD. The pursuit of the magic pill: the overuse of psychotropic medications in children with intellectual and developmental disabilities in the USA. *Epidemiol Psychiatr Sci.* 2019;28(4):365–368.

(35) Uhre CF, Uhre VF, Lønfeldt NN, Pretzmann L, Vangkilde S, Plessen KJ, et al. Systematic review and meta-analysis: Cognitive-behavioral therapy for obsessive-compulsive disorder in children and adolescents. *J Am Acad Child Adolesc Psychiatry.* 2020;59(1):64–77.

(36) Parens E, Johnston J. Controversies concerning the diagnosis and treatment of bipolar disorder in children. *Child Adolesc Psychiatry Ment Health.* 2010;4(1):9.

(37) Mayes SD, Waxmonsky JD, Calhoun SL, Bixler EO. Disruptive mood dysregulation disorder symptoms and association with oppositional defiant and other disorders in a general population child sample. *J Child Adolesc Psychopharmacol.* 2016;26(2):101–106.

(38) Luft MJ, Lamy M, DelBello MP, McNamara RK, Strawn JR. Antidepressant-induced activation in children and adolescents: risk, recognition and management. *Curr Probl Pediatr Adolesc Health Care.* 2018;48(2):50–62.

(39) Mandy W, Roughan L, Skuse D. Three dimensions of oppositionality in autism spectrum disorder. *J Abnorm Child Psychol.* 2014;42(2):291–300.

(40) Noordermeer SDS, Luman M, Weeda WD, Buitelaar JK, Richards JS, Hartman CA, et al. Risk factors for comorbid oppositional defiant disorder in attention-deficit/hyperactivity disorder. *Eur Child Adolesc Psychiatry.* 2017;26(10):1155–1164.

(41) Burke JD, Rowe R, Boylan K. Functional outcomes of child and adolescent ODD symptoms in young adult men. *J Child Psychol Psychiatry.* 2014 Mar;55(3):264–72.

(42) Giupponi G, Giordano G, Maniscalco I, Erbuto D, Berardelli I, Conca A, et al. Suicide risk in attention-deficit/hyperactivity disorder. *Psychiatr Danub.* 2018;30(1):2–10.

(43) Daniel SS, Walsh AK, Goldston DB, Arnold EM, Reboussin BA, Wood FB. Suicidality, school dropout, and reading problems among adolescents. *J Learn Disabil.* 2006;39(6):507–514.

(44) King TL, Milner A, Aitken Z, Karahalios A, Emerson E, Kavanagh AM. Mental health of adolescents: Variations by borderline intellectual functioning and disability. *Eur Child Adolesc Psychiatry*. 2019;28(9):1231–1240.

(45) Shaffer D, Pfeffer CR. Practice parameter for the assessment and treatment of children and adolescents with suicidal behavior. *J Am Acad Child Adolesc Psychiatry*. 2001;40(7):24S–51S.

(46) Carruthers S, Kent R, Hollocks MJ, Simonoff E. Brief report: testing the psychometric properties of the Spence Children's Anxiety Scale (SCAS) and the Screen for Child Anxiety Related Emotional Disorders (SCARED) in autism spectrum disorder. *J Autism Dev Disord*. 2020;50(7):2625–2632.

(47) American Psychiatric Association. *Diagnostic and Statistical Manual of Mental Disorders: DSM-5*. 5th ed. American Psychiatric Association; 2013.

(48) Manassis K, Tannock R, Garland EJ, Minde K, McINNES A, Clark S. The sounds of silence: language, cognition, and anxiety in selective mutism. *J Am Acad Child Adolesc Psychiatry*. 2007;46(9):1187–1195.

(49) Seligman LD, Ollendick TH. Cognitive behavioral therapy for anxiety disorders in youth. *Child Adolesc Psychiatr Clin N Am*. 2011;20(2):217–238.

(50) Hancock KM, Swain J, Hainsworth CJ, Dixon AL, Koo S, Munro K. Acceptance and commitment therapy versus cognitive behavior therapy for children with anxiety: Outcomes of a randomized controlled trial. *J Clin Child Adolesc Psychol*. 2018;47(2):296–311.

(51) Morgan AJ, Rapee RM, Salim A, Goharpey N, Tamir E, McLellan LF, et al. Internet-delivered parenting program for prevention and early intervention of anxiety problems in young children: Randomized controlled trial. *J Am Acad Child Adolesc Psychiatry*. 2017;56(5):417–425.

(52) Wehry AM, Beesdo-Baum K, Hennelly MM, Connolly SD, Strawn JR. Assessment and treatment of anxiety disorders in children and adolescents. *Curr Psychiatry Rep*. 2015;17(7):52.

(53) Jones L, Bellis MA, Wood S, Hughes K, McCoy E, Eckley L, et al. Prevalence and risk of violence against children with disabilities: A systematic review and meta-analysis of observational studies. *Lancet Lond Engl*. 2012;380(9845):899–907.

(54) Collins MSR, Cornish K. A survey of the prevalence of stereotypy, self-injury and aggression in children and young adults with Cri du Chat syndrome. *J Intellect Disabil Res JIDR*. 2002;46(Pt 2):133–140.

(55) Matson JL. *Handbook of Intellectual Disabilities: Integrating Theory, Research, and Practice*. Springer Nature; 2019.

(56) Dudley LL, Johnson C, Barnes RS. Decreasing rumination using a starchy food satiation procedure. *Behav Interv*. 2002;17(1):21–29.

(57) Kozlowska K, Chudleigh C, Cruz C, Lim M, McClure G, Savage B, et al. Psychogenic non-epileptic seizures in children and adolescents: Part I—Diagnostic formulations. *Clin Child Psychol Psychiatry*. 2018;23(1):140–159.

(58) Review: MyCalmBeat | Beacon [Internet]. https://beacon.anu.edu.au/service/mobile/view/41/2

(59) Kozlowska K, Chudleigh C, Cruz C, Lim M, McClure G, Savage B, et al. Psychogenic non-epileptic seizures in children and adolescents: Part II—explanations to families, treatment, and group outcomes. *Clin Child Psychol Psychiatry*. 2018;23(1):160–176.

(60) Santoro SL, Baumer NT, Cornacchia M, Franklin C, Hart SJ, Haugen K, et al. Unexplained regression in Down syndrome: Management of 51 patients in an international patient database. *Am J Med Genet A*. 2022;188(10):3049–3062.

(61) Krefft M, Frydecka D, Adamowski T, Misiak B. From Prader–Willi syndrome to psychosis: Translating parent-of-origin effects into schizophrenia research. *Epigenomics*. 2014;6(6):677–688.

(62) Goldman VE, Naguib MN, Vidmar AP. Anti-obesity medication use in children and adolescents with Prader–Willi syndrome: *Case review and literature search. J Clin Med*. 2021;10(19):4540.

(63) Ng NBH, Low YW, Rajgor DD, Low JM, Lim YY, Loke KY, et al. The effects of glucagon-like peptide (GLP)-1 receptor agonists on weight and glycaemic control in Prader–Willi syndrome: A systematic review. *Clin Endocrinol (Oxf)*. 2022;96(2):144–154.

(64) Horsler K, Oliver C. The behavioural phenotype of Angelman syndrome. *J Intellect Disabil Res JIDR*. 2006;50(Pt 1):33–53.

7

Cases

Cases have been selected to emphasize different aspects of what is discussed throughout the book. In this chapter we reflect on the cases discussed at the end of each chapter and include an additional three cases.

Case 1. Jack

Jack is a boy diagnosed with Foetal Alcohol Spectrum Disorder (FASD) and ADHD. The FASD diagnosis indicates that exposure to alcohol during pregnancy has damaged his brain development, leading to persisting impairments. We have included Jack as an example of behaviour in the context of multiple simultaneous contributing risk factors, each of varying impact. These include his developmental impairments, family, and school factors.

Take-home messages

◆ Jack is not a bad boy. For multiple reasons, he is not able to manage what is expected of him not only with regards to behaviour but more generally across his life with curriculum, life participation, daily living skills, and so on. When he cannot manage, he does not have the capacity to solve problems effectively. His behaviour is his voice.

◆ Jack's past continues to impact his present. This extends beyond the brain damage of maternal alcohol use to include the relationship insecurities of disordered attachment and heightened threat responses that persist after early childhood trauma. To some extent he will carry these through his life. His foster parents need to understand this.

◆ The key to managing Jack is to craft a life where understanding leads to compassion, and compassion leads to effective, sustained adaptations. Jack needs to know with predictable certainty he can be reasonably successful with his endeavours.

◆ Behaviour management needs to be simple, clear, achievable, and reliably sustained. Change will be slow.

- Medication will not fix Jack's behaviour problems. It potentially enables more effective self-control and capacity to learn, but it must be coupled with an adapted environment and effective behavioural management systems.

- The 'therapy' aspect of his care will only be successful when Jack feels safe and ready to help himself.

- Beyond the immediate challenge of Jack's behaviour, the paediatrician is in an important position to support and guide Jack into a successful long-term future.

Case 2. Jade

Jade is a 14-year-old girl in her second year of high school. It is assumed her ASD has a genetic basis given her family history. We included her as the behaviour of teenagers with high-functioning autism can be challenging. It is tempting to collude with others around a subtle 'blame the child' orientation, as youth present as knowing, disrespectful, and intentional. Her behaviour, however, is her way of communicating that she cannot manage life as she currently experiences it.

Take-home messages

- Jade is a challenge. Her quick intelligence and language form a defence against her dealing with the truth of her life. For the paediatrician, the challenge is to find a line that communicates trust and belief in her, avoiding taking what she says personally when she is scathing in her feedback to you.

- Jade is not able to manage life at the moment. Her behaviour is very unlikely to change unless she feels able to manage what is expected and has some control of the process.

- For a seemingly confident, low-insight girl, the proposition that she may have impairments (e.g. as the basis for using medication) may well be very confronting. Such conversations have to be managed very gently.

- A successful path out of her situation needs to be staged. It is reasonable to hold off school attendance, for example, until her sleep cycles and general well-being have recovered. It is a slow, steady, success-based journey with long-term implications beyond her immediate behaviours.

- To re-engage with school she needs to feel safe. Incidents she finds traumatic can set the journey back.

- At all times, Jade needs to feel heard and understood. She needs to participate in treatment goals, strategies, and evaluation of outcomes, and to feel some sense of control.

Case 3. Alfred

Alfred is a boy with Down syndrome and moderate ID. The case description begins at age 5, continuing through to age 15. We included him because the cause of his behaviour was not clear at the outset. This raises the challenge of managing uncertainty due to unresolved questions. Despite the clear nature of his disability, his parents had differing understandings and somewhat unrealistic expectations.

Take-home messages

♦ At the outset, Alfred is an enigma. In this case there is temptation to collapse the uncertainty into a limited and possibly incorrect formulation. It is harder to manage whilst holding uncertainties.

♦ Whilst the problems persist it is important to follow up actively and continuously. As circumstances change and new information emerges, ongoing family support is a critical component of successful management.

♦ In the uncertainty, certain principles remain both true and effective. These include non-judgemental love for the child, efforts to appreciate his experience and perspective, and an environment that is adapted as much as possible to his needs.

♦ To begin with, knowledge of the opinions and actions of Alfred's father was not available. Over time, these became more visible. His inclusion in the decision-making and care over time enabled him to modify his beliefs and parenting behaviours. It is likely that this contributed substantially to the reduction of his son's agitation and problem behaviour.

Case 4. Robbie

Robbie is a 10-year-old boy with intellectual disability (ID). Overall, his developmental skills are around a 4-year-old level, placing him at the lower end of the moderate range of ID.

We include this case because challenging behaviour in this population of children is a common and difficult problem for paediatric care. Snippets of a long and complicated journey of care are presented.

Robbie was referred by his GP because there were concerns by family and school staff about his challenging behaviours. His parents are mainly concerned about his behaviour at school. They often had to pick him up from school because of behaviour. This is the third school Robbie has attended in two years. At his first school, he could get overwhelmed in the playground and throw balls at or hit others. The response was to use a 'time out' room or for Robbie to walk around with the teacher. This was ineffective in altering the behaviour. Robbie had frequent suspensions, including prolonged 20-day suspensions, and following that, a partial return to school for a couple of hours in the morning.

Robbie' parents were also concerned about his behaviour at home. They reported that he frequently kicks the walls (usually leaving a hole) and breaks objects, including seven televisions in one year. He swears frequently and is very resistant to parent directions and requests. They note that 'it's his way or no way' and 'he makes a lot of noise until he gets what he wants'.

When Robbie was 5 years of age age and at preschool, his parents report his behaviours were less severe. They attribute this to what was available; for example he was able to ride bikes. If prevented from riding, however, he would get upset and might let down the tyres.

The parents thought that the most helpful intervention was school-based behaviour therapy and occupational therapy (OT) until this ceased in 2020 with the COVID pandemic. The OT worked on social skills in groups, for example sharing, taking turns, and social communication. They note, however, these interventions led to little sustained difference.

Questions

1. What would you like to know about Robbie's behaviour and likely causes?

2. How would you assess this?

3. What would you like to know about Robbie medically?

Discussion

- You would like to know more about Robbie's behaviour. A structured questionnaire such as the Developmental Behaviour Checklist could provide a description of a broad range of behaviour problems, not just the ones which are currently most prominent in the family's mind.

- You would like to understand the context and motivation behind these behaviours. For this, two approaches are recommended:

  ○ Analysing contextual variation. This considers the question of which behaviours are more likely or less likely to occur in which situations?

  ○ Detail about the 'ABC' of his behaviour—antecedent, behaviour, consequences. What are the immediate 'triggers' and potential 'reinforcers' of his behaviour?

◆ You would like to understand perspectives of those involved, particularly Robbie's family. It is possible that his parents have differing beliefs and management strategies. There are no siblings in this case but if there were, their perspective would also be important to determine. This applies further to other important people in Robbie's world.

◆ Medical investigation has not been undertaken since his initial diagnosis. You would like an updated genetic review.

The Total Behaviour Problem Score is above the 90th percentile for children with moderate or severe ID. It is particularly high for the Teacher version, reflecting worse behaviour at school.

The main contribution to the high scores is the score on the Disruptive subscale reflecting the aggressive and non-compliant behaviour. The score on the Anxiety subscale is also high, reflecting the likely presence of 'internalizing' distressed behaviours. Without using a broad-range psychopathology measure, this might be missed when all the expressed concern is about disruptive behaviour.

Initial information suggests Robbie's behaviour is more likely to occur and is worse when managed by certain teachers who appear to have a more authoritarian style. It is generally triggered when asked to do something he does not want to do, or denied something he wants. He settles more quickly when distracted from the situation and when managed by a teacher he trusts, whose style is less confronting.

Discussion with the family suggests they have struggled to find a common way of managing their son. His mother is described as 'giving way too much' and 'too soft', whereas his father is described as being too 'harsh' and 'strict'.

Table 7.1 Behavioural checklist findings (Robbie)
The Developmental Behaviour Checklist Parent version (DBC-P) was by undertaken by the father. His teacher completed the DBC-T.

Scale	Parent	Teacher
Total Behaviour Problem Score	86	95
Disruptive behaviour	32	45
Self-absorbed behaviour	16	12
Communication disturbance	9	8
Anxiety	16	14
Social relating problems	13	16

Genetic investigation showed that Robbie has a rare *de novo* Chromosome 3 aneuploidy. It is presumed that this is the explanation for his intellectual disability, however it is unclear if this is associated with antisocial behaviour as insufficient cases have been reported.

Questions

1. What are the relevant diagnoses for Robbie?

2. To what extent are these sufficient to explain his behaviour?

3. How would you organize what is known into a diagnostic formulation?

Discussion

Robbie meets criteria for the following diagnoses:

- ID—Moderate

- Chromosome 3 aneuploidy

- Antisocial behaviour, potentially sufficient to warrant a diagnosis of Conduct Disorder (CD)

The ID diagnosis provides information about Robbie's capacity to understand and communicate. It does not explain his behaviour, but it indicates that he is likely to manage socially at the level of his developmental function; specifically, his social comprehension and motivations are likely to fall in the preschool range.

The chromosomal diagnosis assists with communicating the cause and expected permanence of his ID. As a rare finding, however, its relevance to the behaviour is unclear.

A diagnosis of CD communicates that his behavioural pattern is likely to be somewhat entrenched, not easy to modify. It also communicates that the degree of antisocial purpose in his behaviour is disproportionate to his intellectual capacity. However, it may also be seen unhelpfully as judgemental.

Rather than try to understand his situation through diagnoses, a formulation structure may be more helpful.

Predisposing

- Robbie's ID means that he thinks like a preschooler. This includes a developmentally preschool egocentric perspective and frustration when thwarted.

- Robbie's ID limits his capacity to understand and communicate more generally.

- Robbie appears to have a reactive temperament, meaning his frustration tolerance is poor.

- His social empathy is limited. This means he is unlikely to modify his behaviour with information about how it hurts other people.

- There appears to have been little consistent behaviour management input.

Protective

- Robbie has caring parents and a committed school.

Precipitating

- The evidence thus far indicates that the main precipitant is not obtaining what he wants, or being asked to do something that he does not want to do. He responds as a thwarted preschooler.

Perpetuating

- Robbie's behaviour is more likely to persist when he is confronted and when he experiences behaviour management strategy as constraining what he is doing.

Palliating

- His behaviour settles more quickly when gently relocated to a calm-down room, or given the opportunity to walk with a teacher he likes and trusts.

Robbie has had a trial of risperidone which increased to 2 mg/day. The goal is to try to reduce his reactivity when he gets upset. You recommend a strategy at home based on preschool level methods and incentives.

A year later

Robbie's mother said they tried a star chart reward programme earlier that year, but that Robbie tore it down and that it had short-term benefit.

You had recommended a professional skilled in behaviour management for children with ID. They received 2 months of support, however there remain significant challenges with ensuring continuity of behavioural services that address Robbie needs.

His medication led to substantial weight gain. The risperidone was ceased and replaced with aripiprazole 10 mg mane which led to improvement in behaviour in that he was considerably calmer, but still caused weight gain.

With regards to expected behaviour, Robbie' parents described the need for Robbie to be 'good', and that duration of desired behaviours (e.g. no swearing/

spitting) may span a whole week. With regards to rewards, an example was going to the hardware store with his father, something they both like to do. This activity was not always linked to behaviour, however, occurring at other times as well. This reduces the association and effectiveness of the reward in Robbie's mind. Another example reward was purchasing a desired massage tool. The time connection with behaviour and reward was the end of the fortnight.

It is your interpretation that both the goals and desired behaviour are not well defined, such that Robbie is unlikely to understand and remember them. There has been little consistency between home and school regarding expected behaviour, and rewards used to reinforce that behaviour. It is likely that Robbie does not make the connection between delayed rewards and the behaviour.

How might the reward programme be optimized?

The key determinants of successful behavioural strategy are summarized in Chapter 5, Table 5.1. Strategy needs to be in line with each of these seven steps, consistent at home (between parents) and consistent between home and school. If the frequency and duration of your meetings with the family and school does not ensure each of these seven key points, the family will need the support of a professional who is able to work more closely with them.

Six months later

Robbie is now 12 years of age and continues to attend a special school for children with intellectual disability and behaviour problems. Unfortunately, Robbie' behaviour has deteriorated over the past few months, becoming more physically violent.

From the school's perspective, this behaviour presents a serious risk to students and teachers. Policy-based duty of care to students and staff has led to a 20-day suspension. At the time of your consultation, Robbie is halfway through this time. His school struggled with this decision as they are keen to care for Robbie. Your conversation with them made it clear you understood their position, empathized with the challenge and workload presented by Robbie, and laid a foundation for ongoing collaboration.

Behavioural triggers at school include the close proximity of other students, and not getting his own way. Data monitoring shows that some days are characterized by high levels of a range of behaviours, while other days may be mostly without significant distress. Some days he is tired/sleepy. The days on which distressed behaviours occur are common: once to twice a week in recent weeks.

School staff have learned when more disruptive behaviour is more likely to occur. Early warning signs may include starting to tear his clothes and shouting out. This can escalate and may include removal of his clothes, defecating, pushing or throwing heavy items of furniture, and threats of violence to staff, for example repeatedly saying 'I'm going to kill you/him'. He has at these times picked up a pencil, but hasn't taken any action at school on other occasions. Staff manage the environment very carefully to ensure sharp objects such as scissors are not accessible.

When staff consider that Robbie needs to go to the breakout area, he has at times charged the gate for 45 minutes. On another occasion, he picked up and threw a refrigerator and tipped over a teacher's desk.

His behaviour at home is also difficult. Again, it is triggered by disagreements and more likely when Robbie is tired. Robbie also threatens to kill his father, who has had to reduce work hours to care for his son. His father attends interviews, but not Robbie's mother who is still working.

One year later

Robbie is almost 13 years old. His mother attended an interview for the first time in 18 months. She reveals that when Robbie is suspended, his grandmother comes to the house to look after him so his father can go to work. Robbie's grandmother is his favourite person. His behaviour with her is much better than his behaviour with his parents. It is very likely that Robbie experiences this as a reward for suspension. The behaviour plan is modified to use time with grandmother as a reward only when Robbie does not hit anyone at school.

Given problems with weight gain from the antipsychotics, a trial of intermittent (prn) antipsychotic rather than regular antipsychotic is commenced. Olanzapine 5 mg prn is administered at school, after ensuring sufficient safety and accountability. The school reports this predictably calms him for the day from 20 minutes after administration. This has led to fewer suspensions.

Key messages

From the outset, Robbie's behaviour has been difficult to understand and manage. Useful information can be obtained when the time is taken to listen to all key people in his world, involving them all in ongoing management.

◆ Pay careful attention to all elements of the seven steps to a successful reward programme.

◆ If something doesn't make sense, continue to explore. In Robbie's case, the connection between bad behaviour, suspension, and time with his grandmother only became apparent several years into care.

◆ Empathy for the school's situation is helpful in encouraging acceptance of your suggestions. They deal with difficult behaviour on a daily basis, with the risk of fatigue for both effort and compassion.

◆ Needs-based (prn) rather than regular medication can be a useful strategy to achieve the necessary benefit whilst minimizing side effects. Those who know the child well can be trusted to determine risk situations and use this strategy wisely.

◆ Find out as much as reasonably possible about the child's brain function, including genetic influences, even if it does not change management with the current state of knowledge.

Case 5. Lydia

Lydia is a 5-year-old girl with cerebral palsy (spastic quadriplegia, Gross Motor Function Classification System (GMFCS) level 3). She was one of non-identical twins born with extreme prematurity. Her twin brother died in the neonatal period and Lydia had complications of prematurity, including intraventricular haemorrhage. Lydia's diagnosis of cerebral palsy was made in infancy. She requires a wheelchair for mobility, and has a stander and braces (ankle foot orthoses (AFO)). She wears glasses but her vision is satisfactory. She does not have seizures and she is on no medications. Her speech is dysarthric but she talks in complete sentences, fully intelligible to her parents. Lydia is receiving speech therapy and physical therapy. She is independent in her wheelchair, has fair fine motor function, but writing is difficult. It is presumed her cognitive capacity falls within the normal range.

We include her as a case example because her behaviour itself is not particularly disruptive, however it reflects significant psychological distress. Her behaviour arises from the combination of an anxious temperament and struggles due to her CP.

Lydia was referred because of sleep problems and increasing school refusal. She has difficulty settling for sleep, and usually sleeps in her parents' bed. They carry her asleep to her own bed, but she wakes up and cries most nights, saying 'I'm scared', and she usually ends up back in her parents' bed.

Lydia recently started kindergarten, triggering onset of distress and school refusal. The teacher appears to be providing appropriate reassurance and support, but Lydia sometimes escalates to the point of vomiting. When this occurs, Lydia's mother is called and has on occasion taken Lydia home.

Questions

1. How are these behaviours a problem for Lydia as well as her family?

2. What would you consider are the possible causes of her current behaviours?

Discussion

- Her sleep problems are stressful for parents. If her parents are struggling, this is a problem for her.

- Both she and her working parents are not getting enough sleep.

- Her crying and school refusal reflect significant distress. They are also a barrier to her participation and enjoyment of school.

- For a girl with CP, there may be medical causes of her sleep problems, such as painful neuromuscular spasms and gastroesophageal reflux.

- The combination of sleep onset problems, night-time awakenings, and school refusal around the time of kindergarten entry suggest separation anxiety, potentially on the background of a sensitive, anxious temperament.

- Fatigue from sleep deprivation may be worsening the anxiety of school entry.

- It is possible her early childhood experiences predisposed both parents and child to higher than normal levels of anxiety when presented with new challenges.

Follow-up visit

Your history and examination reveals no evidence for gastrointestinal or reflux-based problems. Further enquiry about her sleep reveals that Lydia is easily fatigued, most likely due to living with CP. She still takes a short nap most afternoons. After a bed-time routine and story, her father puts her to bed, but most nights she cries for several minutes until her mother comes to soothe her. This pattern of behaviour goes on for up to an hour, at which time her mother usually lies down with her in her parents' bed.

This pattern of sleep onset delay is likely to be maintained by conditioned 'sleep associations'. Specifically, her inability to settle herself to sleep is rewarded by being held and soothed to sleep in parents' bed. When she wakes in the night in her own bed, she wants those familiar comforts. To ensure his own sleep, Lydia's father, who works long hours, picks her up and brings her back to their bed, where she quickly falls asleep. In this way, her pattern of behaviour is reinforced.

Her parents confirm that Lydia has always had a sensitive temperament that easily escalates into anxiety. They describe this as common in their family.

Regarding early childhood impact, Lydia's mother tearfully acknowledges that she is very anxious about Lydia starting kindergarten, adding 'I am afraid of losing her too'. You take the opportunity to explore unresolved grief and the heightened anxiety of the mother–child dyad with open-ended questions and reflective listening.

You reassure her parents that Lydia's distress and crying at transition to kindergarten is common, and should settle with coordinated support from family and school. Her parents agree to continue working with the teacher on implementing supports and strategies in school to make the transition as gentle as possible for Lydia.

Six months later

You meet again in consultation. Lydia is now aged 6. She makes good eye contact but she does not engage with you in conversation. At home, Lydia is described as talkative and generally happy, easily upset, worrying about everyday issues, and needing repeated reassurance from her parents. She continues to have sleep problems.

Her teachers note that she is now able to transition into kindergarten without undue distress, but she continues to be anxious and socially withdrawn whilst there. She has limited engagement with peers and barely talks with her teacher. The school is concerned because she has much potential but she is not participating. There is no evidence of bullying or other adverse causes.

Questions

1. Lydia does not respond readily to conversational prompts. How can you assess her cognitive and language abilities and social-emotional development? This is to make sure there are no underlying problems in these developmental areas.

2. What other information would you seek to understand this behaviour?

Discussion

If Lydia cooperates without talking, you should be able to administer the Peabody Picture Vocabulary Test, which requires pointing only. This may confirm her strong receptive vocabulary and verbal reasoning. For spoken language, several strategies to observe directly are available: observe family play and interaction in the waiting area; use a clinic observation room with one-way mirror and audio: ask her parents to bring video of interactions at home.

Follow-up visit

From these observations it is clear Lydia has strong language and verbal reasoning. However, her speech intelligibility is impaired by dysarthria, associated with frequent drooling. It is likely that her speech difficulties influence her choice to be silent outside the safety of the family home.

More formal assessment of anxiety includes parent-completed Screen for Childhood Anxiety and Related Disorders (SCARED). Results are consistent with Generalized Anxiety Disorder (GAD) with associated selective mutism. This is consistent with family history as noted above.

In conversation with her teacher, you discuss her individual support plan. The teacher notes that other children had teased her about drooling and speech, causing Lydia significant embarrassment. She is self-conscious, aware of her differences, and this is contributing to her selective mutism and social withdrawal.

With regards to learning, you discuss her problems with fine motor control. Lydia will have problems with handwriting and other manual dexterity tasks. From the outset, this needs to be managed with a variety of strategies, such that she is able to communicate without shame. The school plans to have the special education teacher and an occupational therapist evaluate her further.

Six months later

You are seeing Lydia in the clinic for a follow-up visit. Her parents are seeking guidance regarding sleep. They have made some progress, including eliminating the afternoon nap, establishing with Lydia goals and rewards for going to sleep in her own bed and using a star chart to help monitor and reward her progress.

Their main concern is her anxiety. This is likely to be a lifelong challenge for Lydia. As a result, management is more than responding to problem behaviours. It includes prevention and building Lydia's capacity to understand and manage herself. This requires more than you are able to offer in the clinic setting. You suggest first, a referral for parent training, and second, family therapy to help manage Lydia's anxiety disorder.

Questions

1. It is possible that Lydia's parents interpret these suggestions as indicating you consider them responsible for Lydia's problems. What is the best way to communicate with the parents, and Lydia herself, the purpose of the referrals?

2. What is the best way to undertake these referrals in practice?

3. For Lydia's sleep, what are the potential risks and possible benefits of starting treatment with melatonin?

Discussion

Communicating with the family

After acknowledging the great work they are already doing, the purpose of these referrals is to learn new skills so they are able to manage a sensitive, somewhat challenging child in better ways. This goes beyond management of her current struggles to include prevention and building Lydia's capacity to manage herself. The family is central to these goals.

The purposes of these two referrals are somewhat distinct. Parent training is likely to be relatively structured and manualized, providing and implementing strategies to achieve specific behavioural goals, especially sleep. It may assist the family in the practical aspects of behavioural strategy, such as coordination (between parents) and consistency. The referral for family therapy is directed more at resolution of Lydia's anxiety disorder, so that she is better able to participate in school, and parental grief and loss—both for Lydia's twin brother, and their adjustment to Lydia's disabilities. It is to help the family manage their daughter's emotional health more effectively.

Referral methodology

It is important to select somebody who has the experience and sensitivity to manage Lydia's selective mutism. Where possible, it is helpful to discuss diagnostic presumptions and goals of treatment with the therapist. Similarly, conversation enables the therapist to provide the paediatrician with an understanding of the therapist's likely approach to achieve these goals.

Melatonin

Melatonin may assist with sleep onset, shortening sleep latency (the time between bed-time and falling asleep). It is not likely to help, however, with her night waking behaviours. As both problems are amenable to behavioural interventions, and her parents have some success with this, it may be better to build on their successes with parent training.

Six months later

At review, Lydia's parents report many benefits from parent training (Stepping Stones Triple P). Her sleep problems have largely resolved. However, despite weekly family therapy visits, she continues to have selective mutism and GAD symptoms that interfere with her participation. A parent-completed SCARED shows no substantial change in Lydia's anxiety symptoms. Her parents ask about the use of medication for her anxiety, her mother noting that sertraline had been very helpful to her in managing her own anxiety symptoms.

Questions

1. What are the pros and cons of pharmacotherapy for Lydia's anxiety disorder?

2. If you began treatment, for example with sertraline, how would you measure her response to treatment?

Discussion

Family therapy has helped Lydia's parents understand the interactive nature of separation anxiety, and acknowledge and explore their own experience of grief and loss. Repeat parent-completed SCARED questionnaire shows no substantial change in Lydia's anxiety symptoms. As the impact of anxiety continues despite successful engagement with therapies—and a strong family history of anxiety disorders (responsive to sertraline)—it is reasonable to begin a trial of a Selective Serotonin Reuptake Inhibitor (SSRI) in Lydia. There are no contraindications in the use of SSRIs in children with cerebral palsy or atypical neurodevelopment, but you should use low doses and build dosage cautiously.

When considering achievement of treatment related outcomes, it is important to distinguish behaviours directly driven by anxiety from those that have an alternative cause, such as habituated adaptation. Lydia may not begin to talk to strangers, but may have behaviours that are more socially engaged. She may continue to struggle with sleep onset and night awakenings but the behaviour management of getting her off to sleep, and staying in her own bed, should become easier.

At school, teacher information can monitor willingness to talk and participate. Your own observation will note behaviour in the clinic. For greater objectivity, a regular (e.g. monthly) follow-up parent-completed SCARED, may be beneficial.

Key messages

1. Lydia's challenges with anxiety are likely to arise from causes other than her CP. The impact of anxiety, however, is made worse by her motor impairments which hinder communication, peer relations, social participation, and school function. The combination of anxious temperament with functional impairments compounds the problem.

2. Both her anxiety and motor impairments are lifelong challenges. Care extends beyond management of problems as they arise. It includes prevention and building capacity to manage. This includes family capacity, extending to Lydia's capacity to manage herself.

3. The impact of a difficult perinatal and postnatal experience persists. For both parents, her mother particularly, this continues as a form of recurrent trauma, triggered by situations where her daughter struggles. Anxious responses to parenting challenges elicit anxious responses in Lydia, and vice versa.

Case 6. Andy

Andy is a 6-year-old boy with dual diagnoses of autism (ASD) and ID (severe). He is non-verbal, with limited capacity to use picture-based communication. We include him as the management of behaviour with children like Andy is generally very difficult and imposes a substantial workload on all involved, including the paediatrician. In addition, much of his behaviour is difficult to understand and predict. We tell the story of Andy over time.

Andy attends a Special school. His class currently has two students and two teachers. This follows a year attending the school in kindergarten last year. You are a paediatrician working in a public (government-funded) health clinic. You have seen Andy in the past. For this visit you received a request from the school to assist with Andy's behaviour. His family has agreed to a meeting with the school, undertaken by video teleconference.

Andy's behaviour

Prior to this meeting the school provided a written report about Andy's behaviour. In this report they indicated that Andy has always exhibited challenging behaviours since commencing kindergarten. Teachers described behaviours of crying, screaming frequently, taking his clothes off, and launching himself at staff. A few weeks before the end of last term, his behaviour escalated to the point where an ambulance was called. The teachers report that he was extremely distressed and sobbing, attacking any students or staff who were nearby, and had taken off all his clothes. The teachers found it very difficult to predict when his behaviour is likely to escalate as they have not identified any obvious triggers.

The school initially called the mother, Maria, to come and collect him but his behaviour had been significantly disturbed the night before at home as well and she requested that they call an ambulance. Andy was taken by ambulance to the hospital Emergency Department where he was given clonidine as a sedative and discharged.

Currently the school reports that Andy is generally non-compliant and refuses to attend to tasks. He screams constantly to the point where the class students and teachers need to wear earmuffs in the classroom. They report that Andy uses screaming to express his distress but also to communicate generally.

Andy's development

At 4 years of age, Andy was assessed using the Griffiths scales to have moderate global developmental delay. He has had no further developmental or cognitive assessment. He can follow one-step instructions. He uses visual cards and visual cues to communicate his needs, including to go to the toilet and to have lunch. Recently he actually started to use the word 'toilet' to indicate that he needed to go to the toilet. The teachers believe that his receptive language skills are better than his expressive language skills.

Whilst Andy can follow one-step instructions, he often will not do this. He sometimes runs away and has to be managed with safety in mind. Andy has behaviours the school describes as 'sensory', including mouthing a lot of objects, particularly metal door knobs and other metal things. He is reported as constantly seeking food. Andy has one word, 'wa wa', which he uses to mean a number of different things. Other than this, his expressive language mostly comprises babble and screams. He is often seen to be looking into the corners of the room and laughing. He can move quickly between screaming and crying one minute and then laughing the next. He might sit and do work for a minute or two and then throw work away.

Question

When you talk with the school, what would you like to know about Andy and about the school?

Discussion

Regarding Andy, you would like to know:

- What assessments have been undertaken and what are their results?

- What is his level of function and communication at school?

- It is important to obtain a detailed history of the behaviours, severity, frequency, and context. Information needs to be as objective as possible rather than interpreted by the school staff. Relevant approaches are Contextual Variation and ABC analysis (see Chapter 3).

- What does the school do before and during behavioural episodes? What techniques have been used to address the behaviour and what are the outcomes of those attempts?

- To what extent are Andy's behaviours at school consistent with those reported at home by his mother?

Regarding the school, you would like to know:

- How does the school understand the reasons for Andy's behaviour?

- It is useful to gain an understanding of the school's attitude to Andy. Is the school keen to work with the paediatrician on the problems or does the school want to move him elsewhere?

The school manages his behaviour by giving him preferred tasks and sensory activities to settle. Even when he is settled, they mostly need to work with him on a one to one basis.

Andy's mother Maria reports similar behaviour at home. Andy can be very unpredictable and his behaviour escalates very quickly. She is unable to identify what the triggers are for these escalations. Maria reports that she is generally unable to leave the house with him even to go food shopping. When in the community she finds that people are stopping her to tell Andy to keep quiet. She has needed to call security when he is screaming and distressed. His sensory behaviours are similar at home, including mouthing metal doors, pipes, and cutlery. She reports that if allowed, Andy could sit in the pantry and eat one meal after another.

In general, the school seems sympathetic to Andy's problems and would like to help. They appreciate that similar behaviours occur at home. They find it difficult to know why and predict when he will behave as he does, finding the workload of his day-to-day care very difficult.

Question

What other information would you like to know to understand possible causes of Andy's behaviour?

Discussion

Medical aetiology

Beyond a better explanation for Andy's problems generally, consideration needs to be given to the possibility of a genetic syndrome associated with hyperphagia such as Prader–Willi or Schaaf–Yang syndromes. Given the pica, a lead level is needed.

Behaviour

There is a need to assess from a broad range of perspectives.

- It is useful to obtain a structured account of the problem behaviours, (See Chapter 3), as well as an unstructured history. This will ensure that less prominent but potentially important behaviours will be detected. Also, it will be helpful as a baseline for measuring therapy effects. A simple daily behavioural diary from school may help with this.

- A sensory profile may help understand the extent to which he finds different sensations (sounds, visual, tactile, tastes, smells) problematic.

- A functional behavioural profile may provide information about motivations for behaviour in particular circumstances.

Genetic assessment and investigation did not identify any of these specific syndromes or other conditions. His lead level was not high. There was no history to suggest seizures. The question of medical aetiology remains unresolved.

The sensory profile and functional behaviour analysis added little to what is already known about Andy. Some of his behaviour is predictable (e.g. avoiding situations they know he does not like, responding to loud and sudden noises) but much of it seems to occur for no apparent reason, and for purposes that cannot be understood.

The school has agreed to maintain a daily diary that includes simple structured information of situation (trigger), type, severity, and duration of behaviour.

Questions—diagnosis and formulation

1. At this stage, what diagnoses would you use with Andy?

2. What are the potential limitations of these diagnoses?

3. How would you organize what you know into a formulation to explain Andy's behaviour?

Discussion

Andy's original diagnosis was ASD due to his behaviour and communication. The extent to which this remains central to understanding Andy may have reduced as his behaviour, communication, and social impairments are generally consistent with his intellectual level.

In addition to severe ID, Andy probably qualifies for the DSM-5 label of Unspecified Disruptive, Impulse-Control, and Conduct Disorder (F91.9). Sometimes the most applicable diagnoses are the more non-specific ones available in the ICD-11 or DSM-5.

These diagnoses are descriptive, however, adding little beyond the criteria used to make the diagnosis.

Despite the limitations of what is known, the information available can be organized into a useful formulation structure:

Predisposing

+ Limited comprehension of situations and what is required. This includes social comprehension at or below the developmental level of his cognition and communication (about 18–24 months). Very limited capacity for communication of wants.

+ Fatigue.

+ He becomes upset and agitated when things go wrong and some of his behaviour may be to help himself soothe.

+ He has little to no concept of safety.

Protective

+ Committed mother and school.

Precipitating

+ Being asked to do non-preferred tasks.

+ Otherwise unclear—no pattern to the sensory triggers, context expectations or timing.

Perpetuating

+ Not clear—he seems to get upset and settle largely in his own time.

Palliating

+ Sensory stimulation to soothe.

Eighteen months later

It is 18 months since you have seen Andy and his mother Maria. During this time (the COVID-19 epidemic), the family consulted a private paediatrician but has returned to seek advice from the clinic again.

Maria reported that during and following the lockdown, Andy's behaviour worsened. At home they are variable in frequency and severity, currently worse over the past few weeks. He bangs loudly with spoons on the bench, and often screams, causing the neighbours to complain. Sometimes he runs around naked. If people get too near he pushes them away and tries to attack them. In addition to impact on the family, his behaviour seems to reflect distress for Andy himself. He started head banging and hitting himself. Mother and school feel his behaviour is somewhat worse when he is out of routine. At home and school, Andy still requires constant supervision as he does not have the concept of safety and will frequently abscond.

Andy has developed a behaviour of lying prone on the floor and grinding or thrusting his abdomen at the floor. This can last up to 30 to 60 minutes, several times a day. Sometimes he becomes red in the face. This behaviour is also noted at school.

Maria attributed much of this deterioration in his behaviour to the loss of routines and structure, especially not being able to attend school over the past 3 to 4 months. He is now back at school.

To treat his apparent agitation, Andy has been given several different antipsychotics at different times including risperidone and olanzapine. He is currently taking amisulpride along with clonidine and melatonin at night. These medications have made him a little calmer, however he has gained 12 kilos in weight and is quite obese. In addition to managing Andy's behaviour, Maria would like to change medication in order to alter his significant weight gain. The antipsychotic medication was changed to aripiprazole.

Consideration has been given to causes of the lying on the floor movements. Is it a stereotypy? Is it a dystonia from the antipsychotics? Is it a sensory-seeking behaviour? Is it a pain-related behaviour?

Six months later

Investigations showed that Andy had constipation with faecal impaction and overflow. This was treated with macrogol (polyethylene glycol) supplements. The lying on the floor with abdominal thrusting behaviour then declined, but weight gain continued. Aripiprazole was discontinued with a decision to manage without antipsychotic treatment.

Further follow-up

Andy is now 8 years old. Maria reports that over the last year, with the end of the COVID-19 pandemic, a more predictable routine has been maintained. His behaviour has improved considerably, except when routines have been unavoidably changed such as when his mother spent a period in hospital.

There has been no aggressive behaviour towards others but he continues to hit his chest with his fist. This has caused minor bruising to the chest wall but no apparent other injury. He can still be noisy but not as much as previously. He has lost 15 kilos since ceasing antipsychotics. He continues to take clonidine and melatonin at night.

Question

Has your formulation been modified in light of this information and experience?

Discussion

With better understanding:

- **Precipitating** factors now include constipation and loss of behavioural routine.

- **Palliating** factors now include provision of regular daily routines presented to Andy in visual form so he knows what is happening every day.

Key messages

1. Despite the best initial assessment, the cause of behaviour problems may not be clear. This is particularly true for a child who is unable to communicate their experience and needs.

2. As time and experience provide new information, it is important to modify causal understanding/diagnostic formulation. This is a work in progress, building over time.

3. This process is collaborative with the family. It is similar to science which builds through cycles of hypothesis → prediction → experiment → review → revise.

4. Physical complaints such as reflux and constipation are common causes of behaviour problems in non-verbal children.

5. DSM and ICD include non-specific 'unspecified' diagnoses. These are often appropriate in children with severe disabilities where diagnostic categorisation is required, for example to access services and supports.

6. Even when things are not improving, the value of structured care for families that struggle is likely to be deeply appreciated and ultimately beneficial for the child. At the core of care is a regular collaborative and respectful working relationship with the family.

Index

For the benefit of digital users, indexed terms that span two pages (e.g., 52–53) may, on occasion, appear on only one of those pages.

Note: Tables and figures are indicated by an italic *t* and *f* following the page number.